The Scott, Foresman PROCOM Series

Series Editors

Roderick P. Hart
University of Texas at Austin

Ronald L. Applbaum
Pan American University

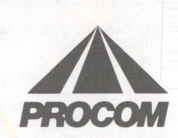

Titles in the PROCOM Series

BETTER WRITING FOR PROFESSIONALS
A Concise Guide
Carol Gelderman

BETWEEN YOU AND ME
The Professional's Guide to Interpersonal Communication
Robert Hopper
In consultation with Lillian Davis

COMMUNICATION STRATEGIES FOR TRIAL ATTORNEYS
K. Phillip Taylor
Raymond W. Buchanan
David U. Strawn

GETTING THE JOB DONE
A Guide to Better Communication for Office Staff
Bonnie M. Johnson
In consultation with Geri Sherman

THE MILITARY OFFICER'S GUIDE TO BETTER COMMUNICATION
L. Brooks Hill
In consultation with Major Michael Gallagher

THE NURSE'S GUIDE TO BETTER COMMUNICATION
Robert E. Carlson
In consultation with Margaret Kidwell Udin and Mary Carlson

THE PHYSICIAN'S GUIDE TO BETTER COMMUNICATION
Barbara F. Sharf
In consultation with Joseph A. Flaherty, M.D.

THE POLICE OFFICER'S GUIDE TO BETTER COMMUNICATION
T. Richard Cheatham
Keith V. Erickson
In consultation with Frank Dyson

PROFESSIONALLY SPEAKING
A Concise Guide
Robert J. Doolittle
In consultation with Thomas Towers

For further information, write to

Professional Publishing Group
Scott, Foresman and Company
1900 East Lake Avenue
Glenview, IL 60025

The Physician's Guide to Better Communication

Barbara F. Sharf, Ph.D.
University of Illinois at Chicago

in consultation with
Joseph A. Flaherty, M.D.
University of Illinois at Chicago

Scott, Foresman and Company **Glenview, Illinois**
Dallas, Texas   Oakland, New Jersey   Palo Alto, California
Tucker, Georgia   London

Library of Congress Cataloging in Publication Data
Sharf, Barbara F.
  The physician's guide to better communication.

  (PROCOM series)
  Bibliography: p.
  Includes index.
  1. Physician and patient. 2. Interpersonal communication. I. Flaherty, Joseph A. II. Title.
III. Series. [DNLM: 1. Physician-Patient relations. 2. Professional-Family relations. 3.
Interprofessional relations. 4. Communication. W 62 S531p]
R727.3.S476   1984   610.69'6   83-14018
ISBN 0-673-15559-5

CONTENTS

FOREWORD   *vii*

PREFACE   *ix*

CHAPTER 1

Communication: Instrument of Medical Practice   1

One Cannot Not Communicate   *2*
Why Improve Communication?   *2*
What Will Improved Communication Accomplish?   *4*
Basic Communication Skills   *6*
Summary   *10*   References   *10*

CHAPTER 2

Communicating with Patients   11

Attitude: Patient and Physician Postures   *12*
What a Difference a Word Makes: Using and Misusing Language   *15*
How Relationships Look, Sound, and Feel: Nonverbal
    Communication   *18*
Giving Support   *23*
Summary   *25*   References   *26*

CHAPTER 3

Communicating with the Ambulatory Patient   27

Ambulatory Care and Adult-Adult Relationships   *28*
Outpatient Milieu: Environmental Influences on Communication   *29*
Communication in Outpatient Practice   *31*
Persuasion and Healing: Follow-up and Management in the
    Ambulatory Setting   *39*
High Anxiety: Taking a Sexual History   *40*
Medical Interview Self-Assessment Checklist   *43*
Summary   *46*   References   *46*

CHAPTER *4*

Communicating with the Hospitalized Patient   48

Acute Illness   *49*
Bedside Manner   *51*
Giving Information   *55*
Facilitating Patient Support Networks   *58*
When Care Replaces Cure: Communicating with the Severely Ill
   and Dying   *58*
Summary   *60*   References   *61*

CHAPTER *5*

Network Communication: The Patient's Family and Significant Others   62

Connecting with the Family   *64*
The Pediatric Triad: Parent, Pediatric Patient, and Physician   *69*
Communicating with Geriatric Patients   *75*
Communicating with Patient Advocates   *76*
Communicating with Those Outside the "Significant" Network   *77*
Summary   *78*   References   *79*

CHAPTER *6*

Communicating with Other Health Care Professionals   81

Communication Within the Health Care Team   *82*
Group Goals   *83*
Membership Roles   *84*
Leadership   *86*
A Case for Critical Care: Physician-Nurse Communication   *87*
Decision Making   *89*
Norms   *90*
Communication Flow   *92*
Communication Among Physicians   *95*
Instruction as Communication   *99*
Formal Communication: Presentations and Lectures   *102*
Summary   *109*   References   *110*

AFTERWORD   *112*

INDEX   *113*

FOREWORD

This volume is part of a series entitled *ProCom* (Professional Communication), which has been created to bring the very latest thinking about human communication to the attention of working professionals. Busy professionals rarely have time for theoretical writings on communication oriented toward general readers, and the books in the ProCom series have been designed to provide the information they need. This volume and the others in the series focus on what communication scholars have learned recently that might prove useful to professionals, how certain principles of interaction can be applied in concrete situations, and what difference the latest thoughts about communication can make in the lives and careers of professionals.

Most professionals want to improve their communication skills in the context of their unique professional callings. They don't want pie-in-the-sky solutions divorced from the reality of their jobs. And, because they are professionals, they typically distrust uninformed advice offered by uninformed advisors, no matter how well intentioned the advice and the advisors might be.

The books in this series have been carefully adapted to the needs and special circumstances of modern professionals. For example, it becomes obvious that the skills needed by a nurse when communicating with the family of a terminally ill patient will differ markedly from those demanded of an attorney when coaxing crucial testimony out of a reluctant witness. Furthermore, analyzing the nurse's or attorney's experiences will hardly help an engineer explain a new bridge's stress fractures to state legislators, a military officer motivate a group of especially dispirited recruits, or a police officer calm a vicious domestic disturbance. All these situations require a special kind of professional with a special kind of professional training. It is ProCom's intention to supplement that training in the area of communication skills.

Each of the authors of the ProCom volumes has extensively taught, written about, and listened to professionals in his or her area. In addition, the books have profited from the services of area consultants— working professionals who have practical experience with the special kinds of communication problems that confront their co-workers. The authors and the area consultants have collaborated to provide solutions to these vexing problems.

We, the editors of the series, believe that ProCom will treat you well. We believe that you will find no theory-for-the-sake-of-theory here. We believe that you will find a sense of expertise. We believe that you will find the content of the ProCom volumes to be specific rather than general, concrete rather than abstract, applied rather than theoretical. We believe that you will find the examples interesting, the information appropriate, and the applications useful. We believe that you will find the ProCom volumes helpful whether you read them on your own or use them in a workshop. We know that ProCom has brought together the most informed authors and the best analysis and advice possible. We ask you to add your own professional goals and practical experiences so that your human communication holds all the warmth that makes it human and all the clarity that makes it communication.

Roderick P. Hart
University of Texas—Austin

Ronald L. Applbaum
Pan American University

PREFACE

"Communication? Sure, it's an important aspect of a doctor's work. But you don't need to read about it. Mostly, good communication is common sense."
"Formal instruction is really useless in helping physicians learn to relate well with patients and co-workers. It's a talent some folks are born with; either you've got it or you don't."
"True, he's pretty abrasive with people, but he's a damn good doctor."

These quotations represent the views of many medical educators and practicing physicians alike. This book takes an opposite stance. The ability of physicians to communicate well cannot be passed off as unimportant, common sense, or serendipity.

We are not born with an innate skill to communicate, let alone communicate effectively. Communication, the ongoing human activity of conveying meaning through symbols, is learned behavior. Unlike learning to read, compute, or perform an appendectomy, it may be impossible to pinpoint the exact time or way each of us begins to apprehend how to suggest meaning to another or how to interpret another's suggested meaning. The development of interpersonal communication skills is a lifelong process that involves incorporating nuances outside our own awareness and learning from both informal lessons while interacting socially with family, friends, and role models, and from formal instruction about theory and practice. This book explores all three levels of learning.

Just as some untrained people show talent in music or mathematics, a person also may demonstrate a natural ability for articulating clearly or engendering warm feelings in others. But it is a fallacy to conclude that the person who seems to have an effortless gift for communicating well cannot benefit from increased awareness and effort. It is equally incorrect to assume that an individual who has matured without acquiring ease or grace in relating to others will not improve through exposure to new ideas or advice about communication, *if* that person is open to new learning.

Effective communication may be more crucial to the practice of medicine than to many other professions. Throughout the two years that this book was being written, whenever others learned in casual conversation that I was at work on a book to help physicians improve communication skills, there never failed to be some response that confirmed the need for such a book. It seemed that nearly everyone had a ready anecdote that illustrated a memorable interaction with a doctor. Unfortunately, these unsolicited accounts were typically descriptions of unsatisfactory encounters, some of which I have recounted in this book.

A physician may perform remarkable surgical procedures or make brilliant interpretations of laboratory tests and thus be considered a "good doctor" on the basis of criteria having nothing to do with communication. Conversely, a person who gets along well with others, but who cannot formulate a correct diagnosis or appropriate treatment plan is not a good doctor by anyone's standards. However, as this book argues, proficient communication is not a frill, but a necessary clinical skill that enhances all the attributes of a truly effective, responsible practitioner.

Portions of the book may appear to be common sense, but from time to time people do not perform according to what we all commonly know to be sensible. This past summer, for example, I entered a hospital for surgery. Following admittance paperwork and laboratory tests, I was sent to my room, whereupon a physician who never introduced herself or her function (I never saw her again) came in to take my vital signs and a brief history. I have no doubt she was busy, in a hurry, and wanted to get this mundane job finished quickly. Thus, she attempted to complete both tasks at once, putting a thermometer in my mouth before beginning a series of open-ended questions like "How long ago did you first notice this problem?" The results were comical. When I unsuccessfully tried to answer while keeping my mouth closed, she failed to understand me and asked me several follow-up questions, all of which I had the same difficulty answering. The solution evolved when a friend who had accompanied me and had heard me recite the history to the floor nurse answered in my stead. Don't ask the patient questions while attempting to take her temperature. Common sense? Of course! But as Professor Sune L. Carlson, a member of the Nobel Prize committee, recently remarked, "most important things in life are obvious once you see them" (*Newsweek,* November 1, 1982, p. 75). I hope this book will serve to focus your sight.

Acknowledgments

Many of the ideas included in this book were in various stages of formulation for several years as I read, prepared lectures, studied videotapes of medical students and physicians performing their work with patients, observed family practitioners in their practices in the Twin Cities and rural Minnesota, and experienced life in the complex Health Sciences Center of the University of Illinois at Chicago. Rod Hart and Ron Applbaum had an interesting idea for a book series on professional communication; their invitation for my contribution to ProCom forced those ideas to take definite shape. I thank them and Scott, Foresman and Company for maintaining faith in me even when I was notably behind schedule with my draft.

Many people indirectly, and perhaps unknowingly, added to and influenced my own thinking about communication in medical practice. They include the several generations of medical students and patients whom I have observed during the "Introduction to Clinical Medicine" class at the University of Minnesota and "Introduction to the Patient" class at the University of Illinois College of Medicine at Chicago. Also instructive to me have been my discussions with graduate students and my friend and colleague Barbara Wood during the medical communication seminars sponsored by the Department of Communication and Theatre at the University of Illinois at Chicago. Randy Voeks and Susan Ackerman-Ross have shared my interest in physician-patient interaction for several years; their willingness to share their experiences is much appreciated. My colleagues in Division VIII of the International Communication Association have been continually a source of research findings, a sounding board for talking through new theories and ideas, and, most of all, a terrific support group. Of this group, I wish to single out Paul Arntson, Gregory Carroll, Gary Krebs, Suzanne Kurtz, Barbara Thornton, and especially Don Cassata for their work and camaraderie.

Mort Creditor, Marty Kernis, and Howard Bers in the Executive Dean's Office of the University of Illinois College of Medicine proved to be unusual bosses in that they made it possible for me to carry out my academic pursuits while still functioning as an assistant dean. Without their consent and support, in addition to the hard work of the staff of the Word Processing Center, it is difficult to imagine that this book would have been completed.

Richard Foley and Kathy Sheridan were particularly helpful in talking me through the peculiar problems of writer's block. Richard was also my coauthor for an article that eventually became the basis for Chapter 3 in this book. Several people volunteered their services to read early drafts and supply reactions that proved quite helpful for revisions. They include Patty Keresztes-Nagy, Tom Loesch, and most notably, Marty Kernis who stuck with me through the end, gave incisive commentary, and corrected my grammar and usage. Stephen Brunton,

M.D., also reviewed the finished manuscript and provided many helpful suggestions that are appreciated.

Special gratitude must be given to my colleague, co-writer, and friend, Joe Flaherty. In several years of teaching and research collaboration, Joe's ideas, as well as his own interactions with patients, students, and colleagues, have profoundly influenced my own thinking. In the context of writing this book, he was a thorough and creative critic, as well as a seemingly endless reservoir of clinical examples and anecdotes. His own contributions in the sections on communicating with dying patients, language development in children, and interprofessional communication were finished in a timely and conscientious manner. Furthermore, his wit, enthusiasm, and positive attitude helped counterbalance my feelings of discouragement several times.

Though not directly involved in this project, certain friends helped me keep the rest of my life going while I wrote. Hilda Sharf constantly offered encouragement and volunteer typing services. Margaret Baughman, Deborah Farrier, and Ramona Kellum have been supportive, dependable, and ready to help at the office, and Rosario LoPiccolo and Paula Zerfoss have been steadfast friends no matter what traumas I have experienced.

Finally, this book is dedicated to the three men who have most influenced me: to Carroll C. Arnold, my "academic grandfather," and Robert L. Scott, my "academic father," whose unwavering belief in my ability to think and write has helped me persist in such endeavors; and to Eugene B. Sharf, my actual father, who has supported and respected my every attempt to stretch and mature. He has given of himself to me; this book is but a token of repayment.

B.F.S.

CHAPTER *1*

Communication: Instrument of Medical Practice

After examining a patient who had sustained numbness in the right hand while on vacation, a neurologist ordered spinal X rays and electromyography. He surmised that an arthritic spur had developed in the thirty-two-year-old female patient's neck and that the spur had been aggravated by increased exercise. When the test results indicated more extensive nerve damage than he had at first expected, he became increasingly concerned. He immediately tried to call the patient; finding her absent from work, he telephoned her at home. He described the results of the test and suggested that the next step was a computerized axial tomography (CAT) scan. Depending on those findings, they might also need to consult the chief neurosurgeon. Unsure of what the CAT scan would indicate, he tried to present the test results and explain further diagnostic procedures in an objective, calm fashion, avoiding making any judgments for which he had an incomplete data base.

The patient interpreted the doctor's message in a different way. Why had he bothered to track her down at home rather than call her at work the next day? Did his request for the CAT scan indicate that he suspected a brain tumor? His mention of the neurosurgeon further added to the patient's alarm, as did the cautious tone she heard in the doctor's voice. She considered that his reluctance to venture a diagnosis might be due to insufficient information, but she could not keep from worrying that he might be withholding bad news.

1

This is not an example of an insensitive physician, an overly anxious patient, or poor communication. It is a somewhat typical interaction, elements of which are repeated daily between doctors and patients. Communication and its consequences pervade the practice of medicine. This book will examine how effective communication skills can help you be a better practitioner.

ONE CANNOT NOT COMMUNICATE

Communication is an ongoing process. It is not an act perpetrated by one individual on another. It is meaning created by people, among people, and influenced by language, nonverbal expression, timing, media, and other variables. It is characterized by aspects that are at once purposeful and spontaneous. Even in informal social settings and particularly in professional exchanges as illustrated in the example above, communicators intend to achieve certain ends. *The physician wanted to convey information* as well as carry out a plan of action with the patient. What he had to say was goal oriented. What may not have been as purposeful was his specific choice of words, his tone of voice, or the context in which he spoke with the patient. These elements are often spontaneous and occur without forethought. In other words, the doctor communicated in some ways that were unintended—*the patient misinterpreted his goal and assumed he must be withholding information.*

Ideal communication would result in perfectly shared comprehension; meaning intended would be meaning understood. In reality, meaning is often shared with varying degrees of imperfection, but the term *communication breakdown* is rarely, if ever, totally accurate. In our interactions with people, all words and behaviors may have communicative significance, whether purposeful or not. Within this continual exchange of messages, mistakes in understanding are normal and should be expected. While this book cannot promise to prevent all such problems, it will help explain why many occur, and will provide approaches for resolving them. Instead of trying to give you a completely new set of communication skills, this book will show you how to optimize the skills you have been acquiring and practicing all your life.

WHY IMPROVE COMMUNICATION?

Why should a busy physician spend time improving communication skills? After all, if you can find the time for self-study, shouldn't you instead focus on new disease findings and treatment modes to acquire knowledge and skills that will *really* aid your practice? The retort is simple: Communication is as basic to a practitioner's competence as differential diagnosis, auscultation, or suturing.

An overwhelming percentage of applicants to medical school express strong interest in being part of a "people-centered profession." While an admirable motive in itself, it could also lead one to schools of social work, counseling, education, or the ministry. But medicine, as demonstrated by countless plays, books, television dramas, and soap operas, has the most dramatic appeal of all the people-centered profes- sions. Even after the romantic notions of the media and beginning medical students are set aside, it is a fact that the practicing physician is privy to confidential information about individuals and families, is the bearer of good and bad news, and from time to time makes life-and-death decisions. Doctors see people stripped of clothes, societal roles, and other trappings; they perform invasive procedures and confront anxiety. Doctors counsel, advise, refer, and prescribe. For primary care physi- cians and most specialists alike, interpersonal contact with patients is an essential aspect of medicine.

Because physicians have often been regarded as both professional and social leaders, the need for effective, clear communication with the public has always existed, although it has not always been realized. The fragility of human understanding between doctors and the public has been underscored in recent years by the growing number of govern- mental regulations and the increased frequency and severity of malprac- tice litigation, which include the following:

> A patient was properly awarded $50,000 in a malpractice suit against a physician who performed a parotidectomy on him without his informed consent, a Pennsylvania appellate court ruled. . . . [The] court said that the evidence warranted a determination that the physician did not tell the patient that the parotidectomy differed from the biopsy that was initially planned. (*AMA Citation*, October 15, 1980, pp. 1-2)

> A patient was entitled to $85,000 in damages under the Federal Tort Claims Act for the negligence of a VA physician in not informing him of the risk of severing his sciatic nerve during reconstructive surgery, a federal trial court in Missouri ruled. (*AMA Citation*, December 15, 1980, p. 50)

> [In the case of a patient who eventually suffered total hearing loss as a result of a stapedectomy], there was a material question of fact about whether the physician had fulfilled his duty of reasonable disclosure of available choices with respect to the proposed surgery and of dangers inherent in each, the [Idaho Supreme] Court said. (*AMA Citation*, January 15, 1981, p. 74)

As these examples illustrate, legal suits brought against physicians are based not only on what was or wasn't done, but on what was or wasn't said. One attorney at a major urban hospital estimates that there are approximately one hundred sixty malpractice cases active at his hospital at any one time. Of these, about half the cases are in some way related to the issue of informed consent. Because legal suits are initiated out of frustration as well as perceived damages, he estimates that 30 to 40 percent of the suits could have been avoided had communication between practitioner and patient been better at the start. No wonder the issue of informed consent and diagnostic or treatment procedures is a major interpersonal, as well as ethical, problem.

With the rise in malpractice litigation, the public has learned more about what to expect from medical practice and is more likely to take action when expectations are not met. In general, patients today are better educated than those in prior generations, and have greater awareness of health-related issues, mostly due to extensive news reports. Because of socially generated movements such as patients' rights and self-help groups, a general progression toward more assertive, interactive physician-patient relationships has begun. As patients begin to participate more in their own health care, the role of the doctor must change in response to subtle pressures to speak with patients in different ways.

In addition to the increased emphasis on patient self-care, increasingly complex professional relationships require physicians to improve communication skills. Whether in urban, suburban, or rural practices, physicians are more frequently viewed as members of a "health care system," which increasingly brings them in contact with other health care personnel. Professional teams for patient care often place the doctor in contact with nurses, physician assistants, social workers, dieticians, psychologists, physical therapists, and laboratory technicians. To meet community needs, doctors interact with epidemiologists, health planners, and hospital administrators. Various vehicles of current medical care such as teaching hospitals, group practice, consultations, and health maintenance organizations require frequent exchanges among physicians. Inter- and intraprofessional communication at once enhances and complicates health care delivery.

WHAT WILL IMPROVED COMMUNICATION ACCOMPLISH?

Now that the argument for paying closer attention to communicative behaviors has been made, let's examine how medical practice can benefit from improved communication. Figure 1.1 illustrates the two major communication objectives inherent in patient care.

The first goal is a cooperative relationship that involves the physician and patient, the physician and the patient's significant family

FIGURE 1.1 Communication Goals in Medical Care: Cooperation and Adherence

A cooperative relationship between the physician and the patient, the patient's family and significant friends, and the physician's colleagues is the foundation for developing with the patient an effective treatment that the patient will follow.

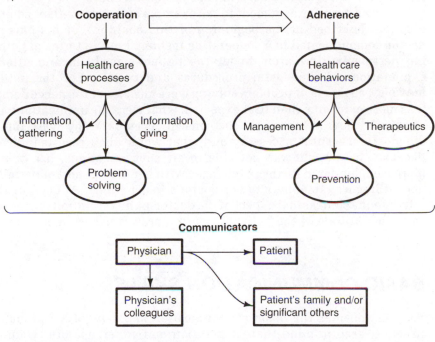

and friends, and the physician and other health care professionals. Cooperation is the communicative mode that is useful in performing processes instrumental to formulating diagnoses and treatment plans. These include *data gathering* during history taking, physical examination, problem listing, and subsequent checkups; *information giving* when speaking at conferences, writing progress notes, and explaining terminology, disease states, and test results; and *problem solving* in eliminating diagnostic hypotheses and considering treatment methods. Cooperating means working together; in performing a task, participants interact and influence one another. When communication tends to be resistant, defensive, or antagonistic rather than cooperative, instrumental health care processes become less effective.

The second goal, adherence, in many ways is an outgrowth of cooperation. Having established a diagnosis and considered treatment, physicians engage in a largely persuasive endeavor to shape the resultant health care behaviors of patients. This effort also may involve the patient's personal network of family, friends, and other health care professionals. Patients must be convinced to accept a *management plan* and follow through on *therapeutic* and *preventive* measures. The model shows adherence as emerging from cooperation since it is more likely that patients will participate in a scheme that they have helped design, rather than one that has been imposed upon them.

Let's return for a moment to the example of doctor-patient communication described at the beginning of this chapter. For his part, the doctor communicated in a cooperative fashion, both in terms of gathering pertinent information about the patient's problem and offering explanations of diagnostic procedures and results. For the patient, however, elements of problem solving were missing: If the nerve damage was more extensive than first expected, what were the implications and, especially, how severe could the consequences be? Why were further diagnostic measures necessary and what would their results indicate? Because the patient was not able to air such questions, her anxiety increased, hindered further exchanges with her doctor, and undermined her willingness to adhere to her doctor's instructions. Adherence thus refers to the contractual aspect of the doctor-patient relationship as well as to the attitude of the patient toward a prescribed regimen.

BASIC COMMUNICATION SKILLS

As you consider the basic communication skills involved in medical practice, keep in mind that cooperation and adherence are two major goals. The fundamental communication skills explained below will be used throughout this book to describe various behaviors designed to achieve these goals and several other objectives.

Situational Analysis

To some degree all of us are aware of our characteristic communicative behaviors, the way we express our ideas, show displeasure or approval, make requests, and so forth. We are, however, less conscious of the full range of alternative behaviors available to us, even though we may occasionally use some of them. Our communication patterns are choices we can make strategically. The choices made in any interpersonal exchange are prompted by the participants, needs, goals, and limitations of that particular situation. Environmental variables such as the setting and sociocultural expectations shape interactions as well. The more we are able to recognize the relevant factors that influence an interpersonal situation and to understand our own range of communicative options, the more we will become effective communicators. This process is called *situational adaptation* and is demonstrated through role flexibility, choice of language, and nonverbal behavior.

Role Flexibility

During a single day, a doctor may have to assume many different professional roles which may include medical practitioner, adviser, supporter, team leader, administrator, teacher, learner, committee member, or public speaker. While certain core characteristics remain constant throughout all situations, other facets will change, reflecting the urgencies, resources, and constraints in a particular event. Certain roles in which we feel less competent or comfortable may cause us to try to disclaim our own performances by saying, "That isn't the *real* me!" Of course it's the real you, but in the context of a less familiar role. The effective communicator develops a range of behaviors and styles that can be used in the various roles required.

Language Choice

One of the most important choices confronting a communicator is selecting what kind of language to use to convey a message. The understood meaning of written or spoken language is generated by what the chosen word denotes—that is, what the explicit definition of the word is —and what the word connotes—that is, what the word suggests or implies. Because connotations may be highly personal and variable, the same word can have different meanings for different people. Ambiguity is built into language use. Being aware of this fact helps us understand, and even expect, that others may attribute different meanings to words that we consider simple, straightforward, and clear. For instance, a recent study compares physician and patient perceptions of commonly used phrases in medical dialogues:

> Apparently when a doctor leaves a patient waiting in an examining room for "just a minute," patients are about three times more likely than their doctors to think that means "thirty seconds to thirty minutes" or even "fifteen minutes to two hours." ("Do You Say What You Mean to Say?" p. 18)

Imagine the differences in meaning that arise when conversation becomes more technical or complex! While it is impossible to plan the exact wording of every conversation you have with a patient, an awareness of the nature of language does show how important it is to choose words carefully and to confirm any apparent need to clarify your meaning, especially when misunderstandings can prove dangerous, for example, when giving instructions to diabetes patients about managing their own diet and medications.

Nonverbal Behavior

Meaning is generated by more than words. In the phone conversation described at the beginning of this chapter, for example, vocal intonation seriously affected the patient's interpretation of the situation. Especially in face-to-face interactions, nonverbal cues convey a great deal of information, both intended and unintended. These nonverbal factors include spatial distance between participants; facial and bodily gestures; posture; paralinguistic or vocal variables such as pitch, tone, and pace; eye contact; touching; and personal-cultural artifacts such as clothing or the way furniture is arranged in a room. Nonverbal communication is probably more ambiguous than language and loaded with cultural and personally idiosyncratic significance. As communicators, we are often less aware of what we are doing nonverbally than what words we are speaking. For this reason, the old adage "actions speak louder than words" may be correct, but it is not always helpful. To look at nonverbal behaviors in isolation can prove pointless or misleading. It is important to be aware of whether a consonance or dissonance between the verbal and nonverbal exists in our own communication and that of others. Discrepancies indicate a need for clarification.

Questioning

Gathering information is a task that is fundamental to most medical care functions. Of course, data may be collected by one individual through reading, testing, or observing. One interpersonal form of information gathering is asking questions. As with the other skills listed here, there is an art to questioning well. How questions are phrased will determine how much and what kind of information is provided. Strategies for pacing and organizing the order in which questions are asked will help define roles and relationships between the participants.

Listening

The necessary complement to questioning is the ability to listen. When significant information is elicited or volunteered, it is often not heard because it falls outside the established mindset of the doctor. This is a common occurrence not only between physician and patient, but among health care professionals as well. Medical training tends to reinforce *critical* listening techniques in which one screens incoming information while simultaneously making judgments. Listening critically while making judgments is a necessary ability, but can have dysfunctional implications for the communication process in some situations. This book will emphasize not critical, but *empathic* listening in which the physician purposefully puts aside critical considerations when relational factors take precedence. In either mode, of course, listening is crucial to eventual understanding.

Organizing

Whether conducting an interview with a patient, discussing a case at a staff conference, or presenting a report at a professional meeting, the way you organize information to be communicated will influence how comprehensible and how interesting you will be to your fellow communicators. Whether to begin in a general fashion and gradually focus audience attention, or to begin in a specific, concrete way and lead to a generalization depends largely on the background of your listeners. Structuring subject matter according to a chronological, spatial, or topical pattern is another choice. Unfortunately, some communicators never seriously consider these issues and instead use idiosyncratic methods of organization that cannot be followed by those they address. Being aware of how you begin, make transitions from one point to another, and end are additional important elements of organizing communication.

Presenting

Once you have determined what information you wish to seek or convey and the way in which you want to organize it, how you present yourself while communicating is crucial. Establishing rapport, demonstrating involvement in the situation, being sensitive to the needs of the other communicators, and displaying appropriate affect (for example, warmth, humor, or sincerity) are examples of presentational aspects. Such variables contribute to your credibility, attractiveness, persuasiveness, and to the quality of your relationships with others.

Discussing

In the process of working toward cooperation and adherence in medical care, there are a number of times the doctor needs to explain, consider alternatives, and make decisions in conjunction with patients, patients' families, and other professionals. In these discussions, techniques for generating ideas, exploring advantages and disadvantages, and advocating a position are fundamental to being an effective communicator. When discussion moves from the context of two people to a group, knowledge of group dynamics becomes useful. For example, getting members of the group to refocus when they have gone off on a tangent, coping with verbose or reticent group members, and keeping the interaction moving toward resolution are common problems that arise during discussions.

Managing

In health care work, it is typical to find physicians in designated leadership positions. Perhaps the most common instance is the management of patients, a responsibility for which doctors have received a great deal of preparation. However, managing an interdisciplinary clinical or research team, or being in charge of a group of medical students and residents are not situations that medical practitioners are necessarily trained to handle during their education. Doctors are often chosen as leaders or managers by virtue of their knowledge of medicine. Understanding the interpersonal aspects of management is expected to be intuitive or is not considered at all. A manager's sensitivity to relationship variables—how information is transmitted among group members, how responsibility is assigned, hidden personal agendas that hinder group productivity—can determine how well a task is accomplished or even whether it is completed at all.

SUMMARY

At the beginning of this chapter a case was presented to illustrate how important communication know-how is to physicians. A communicative framework consisting of goals and skills is one way of viewing medical care functions, in particular those requiring interpersonal exchanges. Cooperation and adherence are the primary communication goals in medical practice. Basic communication skills that predominate in the professional activities of doctors include situational adaptation, role flexibility, language choice, nonverbal behavior choice, questioning, listening, organizing, presenting, discussing, and managing.

In the following chapters we will examine in more detail the communicative problems likely to occur during the course of practice, and some of the ways one can resolve them. This guide is divided according to the particular groups with whom doctors most frequently communicate: ambulatory and hospitalized patients, the patient's network of significant others, allied health professionals, and fellow physicians.

References

Cogan, M. The verdict is in: medical malpractice and informed consent. Presentation at the University of Illinois at Chicago, Health Sciences Center, November 1982.

Do you say what you mean to say? *The New Physician,* 1981, *30,* 18.

CHAPTER 2

Communicating with Patients

A group of students and faculty from our medical college were informally sharing their ideas about the definition of *physician*. As more individuals contributed their opinions, the discussion became increasingly lively. They questioned whether a present-day physician needs to attain computer literacy, but several faculty resisted this suggestion, saying that medicine today like medicine fifty years ago is still more art than science. The head of a large hospital pediatrics department declared vigorously that the most important role of a doctor is and always has been to be a trusted friend to families. A radiologist then reminded the group that he, too, is a physician though he rarely interacts with patients; in the same sentence, however, he affirmed his need to practice sensitivity and empathy with co-workers on a daily basis.

Out of curiosity, we thumbed through the college catalog the next day. We noted that the departmental descriptions of surgery, anesthesiology, and orthopedics tended to emphasize technical skills as well as diagnosis and management. The Department of Medicine proclaimed the physician to be the patient's adviser and the Department of Family Practice stressed the role of patient advocate.

Friend, technical expert, adviser, advocate—these are ways in which doctors describe themselves in relation to their patients. The same qualities are embodied in popular media images that help shape the patient's expectations of what a doctor should be. Think of Marcus Welby, Hawkeye Pierce, and Trapper John. One research team has summarized the purposes of the relationship between doctor and patient as (1) the application of the physician's knowledge and skills to the patient's condition, (2) the expressive interaction dealing with the emotional aspects of the patient's condition and its treatment, and (3) the communication of information (Vuori, Aaku, Aine, Erkko & Johansson 1972). Thus, the term *physician-patient relationship,* which has become widely used over the last decade, is actually a simplified abstraction. When enacted in real life, such relationships are complicated and modified not only by the variety of roles and functions that physicians may assume, but also by such factors as attitude, language, nonverbal communication, and the impact of illness.

ATTITUDE: PATIENT AND PHYSICIAN POSTURES

One tenet of good communication in any situation is to try to assess the attitude of the other participant. Understanding "where the other person is coming from" helps you as a communicator determine the extent of similarity between you and the patient, the sort of resistance to cooperation you can expect, and the most appropriate way to talk with the patient.

Although there are exceptions, one generalization that can be made about patients is that they come to the medical care situation with some degree of anxiety and inhibition. It is likely that the more serious or potentially serious they perceive their conditions to be, the greater the anxiety becomes. Fear and the tendency not to disclose information fully to the doctor stem from the patients' uncertainty about what is wrong with them, as well as perceived differences in status between themselves and you. Though the status difference may be reduced when the patient's educational, cultural, or socioeconomic background resembles the physician's, it never fully disappears. In fact, the separation between patient and physician roles is inherent in the very language we use. The word *physician* signifies a healer and was originally used not only in connection with physical healing, but with those who cured moral and spiritual maladies, thus giving the term an ethical connotation. *Doctor* means a teacher who, by virtue of skill and knowledge, is entitled to express authoritative opinions. Though many professionals have earned the title of doctor, it is most commonly applied to doctors of medicine. Over the centuries, the term *medicine* has been used to refer to aspects of healing, godliness, and magic. *Patient* on the other hand is derived from the roots meaning *later, to suffer,* and *I repent.* A patient has historically been one who is persistent, constant, diligent, able to endure suffering calmly, and is quietly expectant. Furthermore, the patient was to be repentant because illness and sickness originally denoted moral depravity, as well as physical disease. The patient, therefore, was a sinner by virtue of being ill. It is no small wonder that patients have come to feel inferior when relating with doctors.

Given the derivations, it is easy to understand the traditional medical model of interpersonal relationships, represented by a passive, deferential patient acted upon by an authoritative, directive physician. The communication problems inherent in this type of interaction begin when such patients tend to be passive or reticent, contribute little information, and expect the physician to assume all responsibility for treatment and cure. This model also encourages doctors to ignore the contributions patients do attempt to make and to maximize the distance between physician and patient. It is this form of relationship that has been the brunt of much of the criticism leveled at the medical profession.

Today's practitioner should be prepared to deal with rapidly evolving alterations in the traditional model.

> Widespread public education and exposure to media have helped make more of the patient population knowledgeable and sophisticated about a range of subjects and procedures related to health care. Not only are some people capable of understanding a great deal about their health problems if properly explained, they also tend to ask questions and seek further information. Such appropriately responsible behavior is sometimes labeled as suspicious or hostile by physicians because it is a departure from the traditional model.

> Misunderstandings occur when the physician and patient hold very different frames of reference due to differences in cultural background. This issue has become more prevalent with the recent waves of new immigrants from Mexico, Central and South America, and Southeast Asia. Not only do language difficulties complicate communication, but various beliefs about illness, doctors, and treatment quite different from those of Western medicine are often the cause of patients refusing to follow prescribed regimens.

> The growth of self-help groups and attention to alternative health care techniques, such as acupuncture and herbal medicine, indicate new attitudes among patients, ranging from assertiveness to distrust toward physicians. The increasing predilection for patients to take recourse in malpractice suits has replaced the implicit trust that once existed between physicians and patients with a growing adversary tone.

In his celebrated saga, *Anatomy of an Illness* (1979), Norman Cousins represents the vanguard of the "new" breed of patient. Reasoning in opposition to expert medical opinion, Cousins checked himself out of a hospital and prescribed laughter as an antidote to what had been diagnosed as ankylosing spondylitis, a collagen disease of the spine. Despite the degenerative and fatal prognosis, Cousins recovered his health. However, his unconventional treatment was carried out with the consent and under the surveillance of his long-term personal physician. Cousins makes this point several times in his book, emphasizing not only his assertive method of managing his illness, but his gratitude for the cooperation of his doctor. It is unlikely, on the other hand, that Cousins' method, which combines independent patient thinking and research with medical support and authorization, will ever become typical.

By this time, you may be protesting, saying to yourself that physicians also span a wide range of attitudes and aren't all cast in the mold of the traditional model. Certainly individual practitioners vary in degrees of sensitivity and flexibility toward others. Subtle factors in the socialization of doctors, however, influence a general professional stance toward patients.

Much has been written, for example, about the difference between disease and illness. Medical education focuses its students' attention on diagnosis and treatment of *disease,* abnormalities in the structure and function of body organs and systems. Patients focus on *illness,* their subjective experiences of being sick. The two frames of reference do not necessarily correlate. The same disease, organically defined, may be manifested by variously perceived symptoms, pain, and discomfort; feelings of illness may occur without discernable organic disease (Reading 1977). Because of this incongruence, many patients have left encounters with their physicians believing they were treated in a fragmented or aloof manner. That doctors can fall into the trap of treating a disease rather than a person's illness is demonstrated in the hospital ward when doctors talk about "the MI in room 202" or the "renal failure in intensive care."

Perhaps a better example of an unintended attitude toward patients is the frequent use of the term *compliance.* The issue of compliance has recently gained a great deal of attention and is serving as a primary criterion of the effectiveness of medical care. In Chapter 1, the major communicative goals in medical care were identified as *cooperation* in

FIGURE 2.1   *Attitudinal Influences on Physician-Patient Communication*

Assumptions about health care
Cultural background
Educational background
Emphasis on *disease* versus *illness*
Role expectations
Differences in social status

the process of health care and *adherence* to a solution or decision, while the word *compliance* was intentionally avoided. Compliance is distinctly different in that it denotes that one person must act in accordance with the wishes of another; in other words, there is a power relationship implicit in the meaning. To comply with doctor's orders negates the notion that a patient has cooperated in problem solving or has adhered to a plan of his or her own choice. The centrality of compliance as a desired goal evokes the traditional medical model that only the physician, not the patient, is a decision maker in matters concerning the patient's own health.

WHAT A DIFFERENCE A WORD MAKES: USING AND MISUSING LANGUAGE

The aforementioned explanation of how the embedded meanings of the words *physician* and *patient* have implicitly shaped behaviors illustrates the important point that language and our perceptions of reality are inseparable. John McKnight (1980) of the Center for Urban Affairs at Northwestern University argues that Americans have "commodified" the concept of health, at least partially through language use. The original significance of health is a state of wholesomeness and well-being. The word for health in other languages, for example, *salud* in Spanish or *shalom* in Hebrew, signifies conditions even beyond the physical—completeness, peace, and safety. In modern American usage, however, health is conceptualized as a product to be measured, bought, and sold. We speak of the health care industry with physicians as health providers, and patients as health consumers. Of course, health can be neither consumed nor provided, but our terminology has altered our attitudes and approaches to health maintenance and restoration.

Words are the major form of human symbolization. Some social scientists consider the ability to symbolize so important as to be the differentia between humanity and other forms of animal life. Words communicate meaning in two ways. *Denotative* meaning is the literal definition; it is the tangible or intangible thing to which a word refers. Medical doctors are often accused of using unnecessarily complicated jargon, even among themselves. As one practitioner wryly observed in the *New England Journal of Medicine,* "patients ambulate, visualize, articulate, and masticate when the rest of us walk, see, talk, and chew" (Rowland 1979, p. 507). What physicians do not realize is that many patients do not understand vocabulary that doctors assume is commonly known. In one study (Samora, Saunders & Larson 1961) hospitalized patients were asked to define a list of terms that physicians typically used with them. For instance, *appendectomy* denotes "the surgical removal of the appendix vermiformis," but patients thought it to be a cut rectum, sickness, the stomach, an arm or leg, something contagious, something like an epidemic, or something to do with the bowels. Likewise, *respiratory* denotes "pertaining to the act or function of breathing," but was variously reported by the patients to mean dangerous, in the arms, legs, or heart, venereal, resulting from one's work, piles, a sickness in which one sweats and has hot and cold flashes, and tiredness.

In short, patients will substitute vague and inaccurate approximations when they do not know the meaning of words you use. Often they are embarrassed to let you know that they do not understand. Problems in comprehending the nature of illness, the necessity and directions for treatment, or issues of consent stem from these types of situations.

Language also has *connotative* meaning, the subjective significance that resides in the minds of individuals based on their life experiences. Thus, *surgery* commonly denotes the treatment of disease or injury by manual operation. The same word may carry such connotations as painful, unpleasant, terrifying, fascinating, difficult, minor, life-threatening, or life-saving, depending on whether the communicator is surgeon or patient, adult or child, has had surgery personally or knows someone else who has, and a multitude of other factors. Connotations are even more variable and individualized than denotations.

To share intended meaning with patients, physicians must conscientiously make explanations in simple language. It was several days before one patient finally understood the meaning of a question that the hospital staff has asked repeatedly. Why had they asked her if she had "voided," she pointed out, when they could have simply asked her if she had "peed" (Samora et al. 1961).

Physicians also must take the initiative to check frequently with patients about their understanding of key words and phrases that have been discussed with them. In a research project that was designed to ascertain the degree to which patients understood physicians' explanations (Golden & Johnson 1970), investigators talked with patients immediately after they met with the doctors. More than one-third of the patients demonstrated a "significant distortion" in understanding what their doctors had said. As part of the research design, the physicians had the choice of staying to listen to the patient's rendition of their discussion or leaving the room. It is striking to note that in twenty-four of the twenty-five cases, the physician chose to leave, without being asked to do so, before hearing whether the patient had understood clearly.

The traditional model of physician-patient communication assumes a one-way channel. The physician expects that what he or she has told the patient is in itself sufficient and clear. More realistically, communication in medical practice must include *feedback*, whereby the patient is encouraged to summarize and react to what the physician has said. Only in this way can the physician judge whether restatement,

FIGURE 2.2 Traditional Versus Interactional Communication Between Physician and Patient

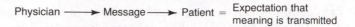

Traditional physician-patient communication

Physician ⟶ Message ⟶ Patient = Expectation that meaning is transmitted

Interactional physician-patient communication

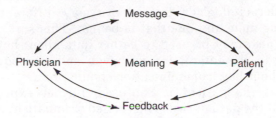

clarification, or additional information is needed. Meaning is not conveyed from one to another, but created as a result of the interaction between the physician and the patient.

Verbal misunderstanding may have comic overtones, as in the case of a woman who had fibroids surgically removed from her uterus. In relating her medical history to a resident, she reported that "fireballs" had been taken out of her "useless." Imagine what images this patient had constructed of her own anatomy and the surgeon's procedure! However, the importance of patients' comprehension of terminology cannot be underestimated, as a letter to the editor of the *New England Journal of Medicine* demonstrates:

Recently my mother died. The death certificate read: "renal failure due to obstruction of the *ureters* by a carcinoma of the ovary." Actually, the true cause of death was considerably more complex. My mother had undergone a total hysterectomy 15 years earlier and, like thousands of other women in America who have been subjected to this operation, thought that all her reproductive organs had been removed.

. . . Women . . . think that the word "hysterectomy" means the surgical removal of all reproductive organs, but the medical community uses the word to indicate the surgical excision of only the womb or uterus. . . .

. . . Because she [the mother] did not fully understand the extent of the operation, she sacrificed any hope of early cancer detection through periodic pelvic examination. (Kane 1979)

HOW RELATIONSHIPS LOOK, SOUND, AND FEEL: NONVERBAL COMMUNICATION

Of course human relationships are defined not only by what is said, but by how things are said. Nonverbal dimensions—interpersonal influences in addition to words—must be considered in medical communication. Physicians are trained to observe certain visual aspects of patients in order to assess possible signs of disease. A slight displacement of facial features, for example, may help detect the occurrence of a minor stroke; a dermatologist's trained eye may differentiate between a precancerous mole and one that is benign. This sort of observational sensitivity also may be used to gather data about how the patient is responding to the interaction with you and, consequently, to make decisions about how communication should proceed. If nonverbal cues suggest that the patient is confused, further explanation may be necessary; if the patient seems distracted or impatient, you may need to interrupt your own line of questioning to find out what is on the patient's mind. A more difficult task is to use the perception of nonverbal factors self-reflexively, to maintain some awareness of your own nonverbal behavior and how it affects your relationship with the patient.

Unlike the meaning that occurs through language, most nonverbal behavior is not a symbol for some external referent or concept. Nonverbal meaning tends to be inherent within the behavior itself. It cannot refer to the past or future as language does; nonverbal significance is in the here-and-now and occurs continuously. Though not mutually exclusive, verbal communication is the main conveyer of content, while nonverbal communication tends to indicate other aspects of the relationship. "Thanks a lot, doctor" is a phrase frequently used by patients as they depart from the office or hospital. This acknowledgment reflects the content of one particular communicative encounter. However, it is the patient's behavior while saying the words that will indicate whether the patient has defined the relationship as adversarial, perfunctory, or friendly. Probably more than language, nonverbal communication is largely connotative and thus is easily misinterpreted. The first step away from an intuitive, random awareness toward a more conscious, organized recognition of nonverbal communication is to identify major sources of nonverbal influences.

The Setting

Physical surroundings, including placement of furniture, extraneous noise, physical and psychological comfort, and even odors, affect the development of interpersonal relationships, sometimes even before the actual encounter between patient and doctor begins. These factors have the potential to increase or decrease patient anxiety, help you appear more approachable or aloof, and discourage or encourage patient disclosures. The next two chapters will elaborate on the specific effects of outpatient and hospital settings.

Proxemics, Eye Contact, and Touch

Proxemics is the study of proximity or how spatial distancing between participants influences communication. The assumption underlying proxemics is that implicit social and cultural rules define our sense of appropriate spacing for various communicative relationships, whether public, social, or intimate. The complexity of medical interactions at times presents interesting contradictions to the usual rules. A physician's concept of professional propriety may dictate a physical distance that seems formal and impersonal while telling a patient the intensely personal news that he or she will die soon. On the other hand, the physical examination requires intrusion into the patient's intimate spatial zone even when the physician and patient, as often happens, are almost total strangers. Being aware of proxemics allows the physician to assess its effects on the patient. In circumstances such as the pelvic, genital, or proctological examination, anticipating the patient's discomfort or anxiety will help you put the patient at ease with an appropriate comment or behavior.

Closely related to proxemics is eye contact, which normally tends to vary with physical distances between communicators. In general, maintaining eye contact is considered an important mode of human exchange. When it is avoided, we tend to feel a sense of alienation, rejection, or even dishonesty from the other person; thus, it is easy to understand why physicians who bury their gazes in notes or in the patient record are not only missing data by ignoring visual cues, but are disconcerting to their patients as well. A patient who avoids looking into the eyes of the doctor may be offering evidence of embarrassment, anxiety, or uncertainty related to a physiological or psychological problem.

An encouraging look from the physician is supportive and can help a patient ask a difficult question or add important information. It is possible, of course, to overdo such behavior. Intense eye contact, outside an intimate relationship, can have the effect of invading the other's personal space and may inhibit, rather than facilitate, verbal interaction. Patients with visible signs of disease or surgical disfigurements may be especially sensitive to the practitioner looking intently. If such gazing is clinical on your part, a concurrent explanation from you ("I'm checking your scar to see how a skin graft could be done") will help alleviate the patient's self-consciousness.

At times an understanding meeting of the eyes is not enough. Nothing short of reaching out may reduce the sense of formal, impersonal distance when a patient needs comfort or support in the face of bad news or pain. In fact, touching is one of the most infrequently used forms of nonverbal communication between physician and patient. Of course, tactile contact is a common occurrence in the very structured activity of physical examination and other procedures, such as drawing blood, administering X rays and anesthesia, and surgery, which may be performed by medical doctors. The uncommon use of touch referred to here is that which communicates affect or helps define the relationship.

In a study of patients and health care professionals in a hospital setting, the results underscored that touching is generally underemployed (Barnett 1972). At one level, this finding is not surprising. In mainstream American culture, touch as a form of social interaction is discouraged. Acceptable instances of touching can be enumerated in short order: the customary handshake or pat on the back, popular dancing, embraces of greeting or farewell, contact sports, and sexual interchange (physical assault, of course, is frequent but unacceptable behavior). But illness, especially serious illness, transforms patients' ordinary social expectations. Infants who are held and caressed thrive and develop significantly better than babies who do not receive such treatment. The desire for this type of basic, preverbal human contact is heightened during the critical points in a person's life, such as serious sickness. Thus, touch—or lack of touch—in the hospital takes on greater importance. In the aforementioned study when tactile contact with patients did take place, it was overwhelmingly performed by nurses and aides; physicians at all levels of training did so the least. In this way, the perceived distance of physicians from patients is upheld. An even more disturbing finding is that all health professionals in the study tended especially to avoid touch with elderly, critically, and fatally ill patients. Tactile separation further alienates and dehumanizes those whose illnesses have set them apart already.

As when making decisions about language choice, you must make judgments about the appropriateness of touch to the individual patient and the particular situation. Naturally you do not want a well-intended gesture to be mistaken for seductive or aggressive behavior. However, sometimes a warm touch or even a humane supporting arm can foster trust or express empathy more eloquently than words. At least two questions are pertinent here: First, what is your own capacity to communicate feeling through touch? Think of your behavior in other contexts with family, friends, and colleagues, circumstances where you are apt to use touch more spontaneously. With conscious effort it is possible to perform some of the same behaviors in professional circumstances. Second, how approachable do your patients believe you are? Think now of how your patients have communicated fear, despair, gratitude, or sadness to you. Of course, patients may extend themselves to you without encouragement, but doctors, by nature of their role, are in a better position to initiate tactile contact.

Facial and Vocal Expression

The most overt nonverbal communication is usually through the face and voice, perhaps because more variety and greater detail is perceivable than in other modes of behavior. Although facial expression is to some degree learned and can be controlled, it still tends to be an indicator of an individual's internal state, in addition to what is said. Furthermore, emotions displayed facially are relatively well recognized and accurately identified, even cross-culturally.

Vocal cues include loudness, pitch, pace, and intonation. Meaning communicated vocally can be separated from the content of talk. It is said that the actor Charles Laughton could bring an audience to the point of tears while reading aloud from the London phone book simply through vocal expression. It is fair to say that a majority of your patients will not have the communicative skills of Laughton, but they still will be able to tell you a great deal, if you are able to listen. Conversely, your own vocal cues can exert important influence. In a study of vocal variables of doctors treating alcoholic patients (Milmoe, Rosenthal, Blane, Chafetz & Wolf 1967), those physicians who were judged to have less angry tones were more successful in referring the alcoholics for further treatment, probably because the patients felt less rejected. Doctors judged to have greater anxiety or nervousness in their voices also were more successful, probably because patients interpreted this tone as showing greater concern.

Both vocal expression and bodily movement, including gait, posture, and gesture, tend to be less self-conscious and controlled than facial activity. Despite proclamations to the contrary, a quivering voice and trembling hands betray nervousness. Due to social norms, patients are often unwilling to express openly a "negative" emotion like anger or disappointment with their physicians, though the feeling is detectable in a brusque vocal tone or a turning away of the body. You may not be happy to hear such negative expressions, but unless you probe the nonverbal cues, there may be unsatisfactorily fixed limits to future cooperation between you and the patient.

An interesting facet of bodily movement that has been demonstrated in videotaped medical interviews is that it may be descriptive not only of the individual participants, but of the entire transaction. The movement of one participant, for example, torso leaning forward or slouched back, legs pointed to the side, or arms crossed in front of the chest, may be reflected by the other, revealing a range of relationship states from empathy to confrontation. The point here is not to plan these nonverbal maneuvers, but to maintain some awareness of them.

Of course, the same principles of communication apply to health practitioners as well as to patients. An attentive patient may well detect a physician's deception about his or her condition even without knowing exactly which subtle cues have given an alert. In fact, anxious or uncertain patients often will be very sensitive to nonverbal communication, noting your let's-get-on-with-it-I-have-a-waiting-room-full-of-people tone which you did not intend to verbalize. Critically or fatally ill patients who are conscious certainly know that the staff is avoiding contact with them. Once again, a self reflexive attitude can be helpful to you in making effective use of nonverbal communication. Videotape is a useful tool for examining your own face, voice, and body behaviors. Feedback from other staff can be helpful as well.

Nonverbal Communication and Culture

Like language, the nonverbal variables that we have reviewed—setting, proxemics, eye contact, touch, facial and vocal expression, and body movement—are subject to cultural variation, making it difficult to interpret such factors in simplistic ways. An Oriental avoiding eye-to-eye contact may be showing deference rather than deviousness or embarrassment. Italians as a group may be more open to touch than those of Scandinavian descent. Middle Easterners may require less personal space than Americans. The research is not complete enough to attempt a classification schema of nonverbal communication according to ethnicity, but depending on the heterogeneity or homogeneity of your patient population, making intercultural distinctions is an issue you may need to investigate further.

Verbal and Nonverbal Communication

Popular literature can lead you to believe that you can learn "to read a person like a book" and that you can decipher "body language." The ambiguity of the nonverbal, in addition to cultural complexities and individual idiosyncrasies, works against such claims. For example, some people play with their hair or beards not out of nervousness, but for unconscious, sensory stimulation! In physician-patient relationships, verbal and nonverbal components usually occur concurrently or within the context of one another. What is important is to focus on interaction between the two modes of communication: How congruent is the language with the behavior? If there are discrepancies between the two, you have reason to probe further. Rather than accept the nonverbal evidence while discounting the spoken, or vice versa, ask the patient to clarify or explain further. Explore affect and check for details of the patient's story until you are satisfied that you understand why the discrepancy occurred.

GIVING SUPPORT

A general aspect of the physician-patient relationship that will be introduced here is the function of the physician as support-giver. Medical education and practice is premised on *cure* as opposed to *care*. Many within the medical profession argue that the public may be expecting too much in perceiving physicians as major providers of care. Reverting back to the terminology used at the beginning of this chapter, the primary framework for the physician is disease. Patients naturally want their diseases to be cured if possible, but they want all the fears and discomforts of their experience of being ill to be attended to as well. Other health professionals—most notably nurses, but also technicians, therapists, pharmacists, and aides—have been trained to help with the process of care, in addition to cure. Also, the patient's network of family and friends may be very significant in the care process. Yet there are still some circumstances in which the physician is relied upon to provide the needed support and attention, especially when confronting anxiety and misfortune.

Coping with Anxiety

We are anxious when we lack information. (How did you feel before you received the results of your board examinations?) Often it is only the doctor who, possessing ample knowledge of the disease, the treatment, and the patient's condition, is able to respond to the patient's questions. Because of the fears conjured up by anxiety, patients may not be able at first to verbalize all the questions that concern them. You must be alert to signs of hesitancy, noncomprehension, or worry which may indicate that the patient needs more information. Since you are not a mind reader and cannot be expected to know intuitively what particular information is being sought, it is helpful to give the patient encouragement and ample opportunity to speak and inquire. Giving support to the anxious patient means helping the patient verbalize troublesome thoughts and feelings, and providing the relevant information when possible.

Coping with Misfortune

The reward of patient care in large part is helping an ill person recover from disease or injury to a healthier state. A harsh reality of medical practice is that such a result is often impossible. Some patients remain chronically ill, but can live productively nonetheless; others never recover satisfactory health. The physician is frequently the bearer of bad tidings, such as declarations of terminal illness, death, paralysis, mental retardation, and the like. At times perception of misfortune is relative and requires understanding and sensitivity to the patient's predicament. For example, announcing a pregnancy to an unwed, teenage girl might seem to her as disastrous as a diagnosis of infertility to a childless, married woman of twenty-nine. Immediacy of the situation is what brings the physician into the supporter role. Communicating relevant information is not necessarily helpful at these times since the patient, or patient's family, may not be in a state to comprehend clearly what is being said. What is primary in this type of situation is to allow individuals an opportunity to express the grief, and possibly anger, that they feel. Your role here is to be a sounding board as well as to offer assurance that honest expression of feeling is not only permissible, but encouraged.

Siegler and Osmond (1979) in describing patienthood make a useful distinction between the sick role and the dying role. The responsibility of the patient in the former role is to do what he or she can to work with health professionals in order to recover; in the latter role, the responsibility is to die the "best" death possible as defined by the individual. While one is in the sick role, cooperation with the physician is usually beneficial and desirable, but the doctor is able to contribute much less to the creation of a good death. The patient's family, friends, spiritual advisors, and nurses can be of greater help. When the physician is needed by the dying patient, it is in the role of friend rather than healer. Much the same is true of the patient who must live with a permanent handicap or impairment. The basic kind of support that a physician can offer when a patient will not recover to full health is a demonstration of empathy, an indication that you will be available if needed, and then deferral to the patient's personal network and other helping professionals who are now in a better position to give assistance.

Support-Giving Skills

Communicative skills that are basic to giving support include *listening* and *empathy*. A recommendation to listen may seem simplistic. After all, you have been listening to other people throughout your career. One problem is that we often do not listen well. Talking with patients, you naturally have an agenda—certain things that you feel are important to pursue, particular tasks that you wish to accomplish. Because of a natural preoccupation with your own agenda, you are less likely to attend to what the patient is saying. Second, many of us have been well-versed in critical listening. Two years of basic science lectures in medical school helped you become an expert on selective perception; that is, you focus on what you determine is important to know and remember, while disregarding what is not significant to you. While critical listening is very useful, even essential, for note-taking and studying, it is not conducive to improving interpersonal relationships. If you are busy differentiating the important from the unimportant, you will not know what is considered important by the other person. Finally, critical listening trains us to make judgments on the basis of small amounts of information. The type of listening recommended here requires that you put aside your judgmental armor until patients have had an uninterrupted opportunity to tell their stories. Ideally, judgments are not made during listening, but afterward.

Empathic skills are closely related and require this interpersonal style of listening. Empathy is often mistaken for sympathy. When we sympathize, we project our own feelings onto another. A patient is going home for Thanksgiving dinner. "That's great," you say, thinking of your own experience with large, congenial family dinners and happy holidays. What you do not realize is that returning home for this patient is aggravating and stressful. Empathy is being able, at a particular time, to put aside your own perspective in order to understand the viewpoint and feelings of the other. It can be demonstrated by "feeding back" or describing to the other person what you have understood after having listened to his or her story. Even when you cannot solve a patient's problem, it is astonishing how therapeutic it is during a critical time for that person to be allowed to express feelings freely, to be listened to in a nonjudgmental manner, and to be understood.

SUMMARY

Chapter 2 has provided an overview of the many factors that influence the physician-patient relationship. Attitudinal variables include role expectations, status and background differences, assumptions about health care, and perspectives on disease and illness. Because denotative and connotative meanings intrinsic to language present numerous opportunities for misunderstanding important information, feedback between doctor and patient is necessary to clarify content. Nonverbal communication—setting, proxemics, eye contact, touch, facial and vocal expression, and bodily movement—may be sufficiently ambiguous to defy literal interpretation, but does provide essential cues about affect and the nature of the relationship. Finally, physicians are sometimes called upon to care for, as well as cure, their patients. To do so effectively, doctors need to cultivate the supportive skills of interpersonal listening and of demonstrating empathy.

The next two chapters will discuss the physician-patient relationship in more detail, as influenced by the ambulatory and hospital settings.

References

Barnett, K. A survey of the current utilization of touch by health team personnel with hospitalized patients. *International Journal of Nursing Studies*, 1972, *9*, 195–209.

Cousins, N. *Anatomy of an illness as perceived by the patient: Reflections on healing and regeneration.* New York: Norton, 1979.

Golden, J. S., & Johnston, G. D. Problems of distortion in doctor-patient communications. *Psychiatry in Medicine*, 1970, *1*, 127-49.

Kane, J. C. Correspondence to the editor. *New England Journal of Medicine*, 1979, *301*, 274.

McKnight, J. Address to the Health Communication Division at the meeting of the International Communication Association, Mexico City, May 1980.

Milmoe, S., Rosenthal, R., Blane, H. T., Chafetz, M. E., & Wolf, I. The doctor's voice: Postdictor of successful referral of alcoholic patients. *Journal of Abnormal Psychology*, 1967, *72*, 78-84.

Reading, A. Illness and disease. *Medical Clinics of North America*, 1977, *61*, 703–10.

Rowland, L. P. Correspondence to the editor. *New England Journal of Medicine*, 1979, *301*, 507.

Samora, J., Saunders, L., & Larson, R. F. Medical vocabulary knowledge among hospital patients. *Journal of Health and Human Behavior*, 1961, *2*, 83–92.

Siegler, M., & Osmond, H. *Patienthood: The act of being a responsible patient.* New York: Macmillan, 1979.

Vuori, H., Aaku, T., Aine, E., Erkko, R., & Johansson, R. Doctor-patient relationship in the light of patients' experiences. *Social Science and Medicine*, 1972, *6*, 723–30.

CHAPTER 3

Communicating with the Ambulatory Patient

If you ever have traveled outside the United States, recall for a moment the first feelings that come over you as you arrive in a foreign airport or train station, or drive over a national border. The faces, odors, and surroundings are unfamiliar and you have no immediate sense of orientation. In many instances, sounds of strange and perhaps incomprehensible language encompass you. An ordinary task, such as asking directions or counting out money for a taxi fare, becomes complicated, time-consuming, and sometimes frustrating. You find you must get help from other people to do simple tasks like using a pay phone or ordering a meal, which at home are done without a second thought. Depending on the circumstances, it can take you hours or days to become accustomed to the new environment. Now, think about your homecoming once you pass the rigmarole of customs back into the United States. Whatever regrets you may have about your trip ending are supplanted by the strong sense of familiarity and control you have in a context you have spent years learning to master. You can carry on your activities independently and at a faster pace. It is comforting to be in one's own environment.

The analogy portrayed here may be imperfect, but the images evoked do point toward differences in the hospitalized and the ambulatory patient, which call for specific interpersonal strategies. People who are admitted to a hospital similarly experience much disorientation and discomfort—as if they were visiting a foreign country. These circumstances create distinct communication concerns that will be discussed in

Chapter 4. This chapter will examine communication appropriate to ambulatory patients, who resemble travelers on their home ground. The degree of comfort, familiarity, and most importantly, *command* one has in an environment will influence greatly the modes, resources, and constraints of interpersonal behavior (Foley & Sharf 1981).

AMBULATORY CARE AND ADULT-ADULT RELATIONSHIPS

Ambulatory care focuses on common nonspecific problems, continuous care of chronic disease, or prevention and health maintenance. It occurs in a variety of outpatient settings, usually in a clinic or office. Contact between practitioners and patients may be ongoing or intermittent. Data generated through communication with the patient often serve as the base upon which subsequent diagnosis and treatment will depend. Discussing treatment procedures or preventive measures with the patient is often crucial to the success of the management plan.

Nearly thirty years ago, two psychiatrists, Szasz and Hollender (1956), brought their understanding of human psychodynamics to bear on the physician-patient relationship. They categorize this relationship in three ways: activity-passivity, guidance-cooperation, and mutual participation. The first two modes are much more suitable to patients treated in the hospital and will be discussed in more detail in Chapter 4. Mutual participation is appropriate to ambulatory patients who can control their own behaviors and living environments. For this reason, Szasz and Hollender use the developmental metaphor "adult-adult" to describe this form of relationship. Chronic conditions (such as those associated with diabetes mellitus, myasthenia gravis, hypertension, or orthopedic problems requiring prostheses) and preventive medicine may require regulating diet, increasing or decreasing physical activity, and administering medication. These are plans of action for which only

FIGURE 3.1   *Physician and Patient as Partners in Health Care*

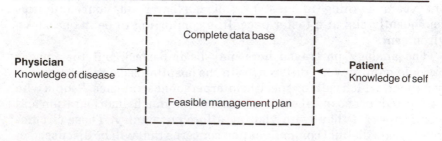

the patient can assume responsibility. Thus, mutual participation presumes the bringing together of two sources of knowledge. Physicians are the experts on disease, while patients are the experts on themselves, their life-styles, strengths, and limitations. Devising a long-term prevention or treatment plan that is feasible and likely to be followed by a patient who is not under the close supervision possible in a hospital requires the patient to be acknowledged as a choice-making adult who is "a full-fledged partner in the management of his [or her] own health" (Szasz & Hollender 1956).

Children, of course, represent a different subcategory of outpatient that does not fit the adult-adult model of functioning. Special considerations for communicating with children and parents will be addressed in Chapter 5.

OUTPATIENT MILIEU: ENVIRONMENTAL INFLUENCES ON COMMUNICATION

In most instances, the patient's first introduction to you is your practice environment. While it is true that your personal interaction is the key factor in the relationships you develop with patients, the setting gives an initial impression, establishes an atmosphere or mood, and helps shape the interchanges that take place. Although parts of the environment may be beyond your control if you practice in a large group or institution, other features are the result of choices you can make.

You can show respect for your patients and acknowledge their individuality by paying attention to basic office procedures. The waiting room office or clinic is, of course, a public space that patients must share. Some practices have supplemented the usual supply of magazines with videotapes, filmstrips, slides, and other instructional materials for patient education in order to maximize the usefulness of time spent in the waiting room. Patients should not be asked by office or clinic staff to relate portions of their histories or state the purpose of their visit in front of other patients. Perhaps what is most important is to avoid making patients wait unnecessarily. The implicit message communicated by perpetually "stacking patients" in the reception area is that your time is valuable, but theirs is not. Visiting the doctor usually requires patients to take time off from work or arrange for a babysitter; their appointments should be treated seriously and physicians should try to meet them. If you have been detained unexpectedly by an emergency, on hospital rounds, or in surgery, most of your patients will understand and accept a sincere apology and brief explanation. Unfortunately, long waits for the doctor have become so commonplace that often an explanation is not even offered. When it becomes clear that a delay will set all appointments off schedule, your office staff should telephone as many patients as possible so they can adjust their agendas accordingly. Such basic considerations set the tone for the more serious aspects of the physician-patient relationship.

Once the patient leaves the reception area and enters the office or examining room, the patient is getting closer to the destination—to be seen by you. It is efficient and helpful for a nurse or physician's assistant to see the patient first in order to perform such preliminary procedures as taking the patient's temperature and blood pressure, or recording certain aspects of the presenting problem and history. However, the process of history taking should be worked out carefully so that the information collected by someone else can be relayed to you in a comprehensible and simple fashion. Too frequently background data gathered in advance of the talk with the doctor is ignored during the interview so that patients find themselves being asked to repeat. Also, remember that the patient has come primarily to see you. Allied health professionals should give a clear statement of their function so that patients will not feel as if they are being passed on to someone with credentials less than those of the physician. For the same reason, patients should not be pressured to disclose intricate or highly personal material that they wish to discuss only with you.

Perhaps the only thing worse than a long stay in the waiting room is being left unattended in the examining room for a lengthy period. Usually the seating for the patient is less comfortable than in the outer office and the setting tends to be sterile and austere, thus heightening feelings of uncertainty and tension. When patients are asked to remove their clothing and drape themselves with a sheet or put on a hospital dressing gown, psychological discomfort is increased and may even be physical as well if the temperature is too cool. Even though you may be accustomed to seeing patients in various states of undress, most people are not at ease initiating interaction in that manner. Thus, it is preferable for patients to remain in street clothes until you first have talked with them about the reason for their visit and background information.

A different sort of environmental factor that influences the communication is seating arrangements and placement of other furniture. How is your office laid out? Are patients seated to your side or directly across from you with a desk in between? In many professional milieus, whether consciously or not, desks are used as symbols of power. Not only does a desk create distance between the person behind it and in front of it, it can aggrandize its user as well. Purposely seating a patient to your side so that there is no obstacle between the two of you helps decrease the sense of hierarchy and separation. Furthermore, a cater-corner seating arrangement encourages more open, relaxed communication; when individuals are seated directly across from one another, the feeling is more stiff and confrontational.

It is important to be aware of differences in seating height as well, which is most immediately apparent when pediatric patients are

FIGURE 3.2 *Environment Influences Communication with Patients*

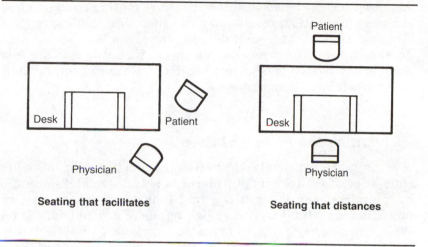

Seating that facilitates   Seating that distances

involved. Not only are children sometimes ignored in a medical interview when a parent is present, but they are symbolically left out when their eye level is significantly lower than that of the adults conversing around them. This problem can be solved by permitting small children to sit on parents' laps or on the examining table. The converse problem can arise when an adult patient is seated on the examining table looking down on the physician seated in a low chair; in this instance, eye contact is interrupted and the patient may feel on display. An adjustable stool for the physician may be helpful, but it is probably a better idea to have the patient sit in a comfortable chair for any lengthy conversations.

Each of the details discussed here may seem of limited importance, but together they form the basis for a considerate, encouraging, and warm environment that is conducive to better communication between physicians and patients.

COMMUNICATION IN OUTPATIENT PRACTICE

Whatever degree of proficiency in talking with patients you have developed is most probably intuitive, based on your own experiences and the observations of more experienced practitioners. However, even for the most skilled medical communicators, large case loads and time pressures have a way of encouraging short cuts and oversights that detract from both the content and relationship aspects of the medical interview.

The following section will examine closely the interpersonal behaviors that occur once your encounter with the patient begins. The major aspects of the medical interview are putting the patient at ease, eliciting information, maintaining direction, maintaining rapport, and bringing closure. The essential guidelines for good communication developed here do not require you to sacrifice efficiency for interpersonal effectiveness; maximizing the data base goes hand in hand with being sensitive to human needs.

Putting the Patient at Ease

Any anxiety patients may be feeling about their ailments when they enter a doctor's office is amplified when they must relate information to a busy professional. When it is a first-time or infrequent visit and the physician is a stranger, it may be even more difficult for the patient. While physicians cannot be expected to devote a great deal of time to patient anxieties, a few amenities can go a long way toward increasing patient comfort.

The first minute inside the physician's office can establish a sense of beginning trust or distance. Patients like to be acknowledged as individuals. Too frequently the patient is not addressed by name or the doctor neglects to introduce himself or herself. Another common occurrence is for the physician to say, "Hi, I am Dr. Stone. What brings you here today, Barbara?" Obviously there is an inequality symbolized in the phrasing and a great deal of presumption in assuming it is permissible to address the patient on a first-name basis. Simple courtesies such as asking new patients how they would like to be addressed and introducing yourself to them (simply wearing a name tag is not enough), or making a reference to the previous visit with an ongoing patient can help establish trust and put the patient at ease.

We have discussed the importance of comfort in seating arrangements. Even more essential is ensuring a sense of privacy when you talk with patients. Remembering to close the door or draw the curtain can create a private setting, even in a crowded clinic. Establishing office procedures to eliminate interruptions by the phone or office staff will provide privacy and continuity in your communications with patients. There is a verbal component to the creation of privacy as well. Patients should be assured that the information they relay to you will be treated as confidential and will not be released without their permission.

Expectations is a subject rarely mentioned at the start of a patient's visit, let alone explicitly discussed. Questions about fee schedules and the extent to which the patient hopes you can help with his or her problems are the two most important matters to get out in the open quickly. When patients see that you are willing to approach and deal directly with these sensitive issues, a tone is set for the remainder of the encounter. The importance of putting the patient at ease should not be underrated, for once rapport is initially developed, a patient's trust in diagnosis and treatment is more likely to follow.

Eliciting Information

The conjoint model of physician-patient interaction described in Chapter 2 showed that both patient and physician contribute information that is central to solving medical problems. The trouble in actual practice is that physicians too often impose their own frames of reference before letting patients relate concerns from their own perspectives. What is occasionally forgotten by practitioners is that by encouraging the patient to describe instead of trying to deduce by "leading" the interview, a richer explanation of the problem is elicited. A good rule of thumb whenever patients present a new problem is to allow them at least ten minutes to tell the story in their own words. For a patient returning for follow-up on a previously discussed problem, the same technique still should be used, but for less time.

Asking open-ended questions is likely to produce the broadest amount of patient information. For example, the patient who complains of diarrhea reveals a symptom that may immediately trigger from the physician a series of questions related to issues such as diet, exercise, and frequency of bowel movements. While these are natural follow-up probes, they are not context specific. One open-ended question like "Why do you think you now have diarrhea?" might result in the patient telling you he or she has just returned from Mexico, or has begun drinking whole milk, which would lead you, as interviewer, to ask more economical and meaningful follow-up queries. Even if the question results in answers that are not highly credible in a medical sense, such as "I've been taking too many aspirin," you obtain valuable information about the patient's habits, level of concern, fears, and sophistication about his or her symptoms. Most importantly, this type of inquiry shows that you think the patient's ideas are significant and that you believe that the two of you must collaborate in a mutual effort to discover the source of distress.

Sometimes when patients are asked, "What do you think is wrong?" they are liable to reply, "That's your job to tell me; that's why I'm seeing you," an answer that stems in part from patients being accustomed to taking a passive role in medical care. Also, this reply reduces their risk of possibly appearing foolish in front of the doctor. One way of avoiding this problem is to ask instead, "What do you tell your friends about your illness?" (Pendleton 1982).

Of course it is impractical or inappropriate to conduct an entire interview with only open-ended questions. Specific queries are needed to probe for more explicit meanings or to clarify data. If a patient reports that he or she is a moderate drinker, you probably will have little idea what this means unless you find out how much alcohol is consumed per day, in what contexts, and with what results. On the other hand, too many closed questions may take more time, yield less valuable data, and even direct the course of the interview down a misleading path. In general, begin discussing every new symptom with an open-ended question. Ask the patient to describe the pain before asking whether it is sharp, dull, or throbbing. The patient may give a description that you could not have anticipated, and which is more helpful for solving the problem. If the patient is truly at a loss for words, however, offering a choice of possible responses can prove useful in getting some sort of description or helping the patient formulate an answer.

We already have discussed the tendency of physicians to use jargon that is incomprehensible to many lay people. Any disease, procedure, or treatment can be explained in everyday language. One way to determine whether you have been clear during the interview is to ask your patients to explain in their own words the information you have provided. Asking to hear the patient's understanding of his or her illness and treatment plan will help clear up misconceptions and provide a forum for negotiating differences in thinking between physician and patient (Stoeckle & Barsky 1980).

In addition to being conscious of your choice of words, also watch certain verbal responses that may connote a very different message than you intended. In conducting a review of systems, for example, physicians frequently go through a mental checklist which is verbalized by a string of okays or uh-huhs. A patient can mistakenly interpret these as signs of approval, boredom, preoccupation, or even a brush-off.

Paying attention to the order and phrasing of questions, your choice of words, and the perspective a patient brings is a technique that elicits a more comprehensive and relevant data base.

Maintaining Direction

Among the most difficult communicative skills is learning to strike a balance between eliciting the richest information possible and maintaining the direction of the interview in order to collect certain kinds of data within the time available. Coping with time constraints, directing the flow of the conversation, determining which topics will be discussed at what points, as well as intervening with a verbose or reticent patient are specific aspects of the medical interview that require the physician to exert control. A few reminders follow to help you become more conscious of these issues.

The pace at which the doctor proceeds bespeaks an attitude about the interaction. A brusque, rapid-fire interview discourages most patients from feeling free to discuss their concerns. A very leisurely pace, in contrast, may give the impression that a patient is welcome to ramble with no limits.

One way to modulate the tendency to move along too quickly, which also provides clarity during the interview, is to use periodic summaries. There are natural segments in the medical interview, such as the chief complaint, history, and review of systems. First, alert the patient to what portion of the interview is going to be discussed; without a brief explanation from you, a patient with severe back pain, for example, may be confused about why you are taking time to discuss previous hospitalizations or to inquire about chest pain or shortness of breath. Then be sure to conclude that segment with a summary of the important points as you understand them. This creates a sense of order and shared meaning of the interchange for you and the patient, indicates that you are in control, and lets the patient know the logic of the sequence you are following. Intermittent summaries and transition statements permit the patient to correct inaccuracies in data gathering and to add information, and also provide some "psychological breathing spaces" during the interview.

Individual patients also will influence the degree of control a physician must consciously exert during an interview. While doctors often are faulted for not having the time to hear patients out, a genuinely attentive interviewer may be confronted by the verbose person who would like to use the time for catharsis or psychotherapy. In these cases, one strategy is to redirect tactfully, yet firmly, the patient's discussion by interrupting with more relevant questions. Another is to say, "We have to move on in order to cover the many questions I have."

A contrasting situation is the shy patient who has difficulty talking, especially about fears, intimacy, or anxiety. Although lulls in conversation often are viewed as a waste of time, they can be used constructively. Merely pausing for a few moments will encourage certain patients to release what is on their minds as opposed to your filling silences as a means of rescuing the interview.

Maintaining direction during the medical interview should not be equated with dominating the conversation and does not contradict the spirit of collaboration inherent in the adult-adult relationship model. It is a way of facilitating the doctor-patient interaction in an orderly, comprehensible, and economic fashion.

Maintaining Rapport

Briefly stated, the major components of maintaining rapport are being attentive, allowing the patient freedom of expression, minimizing anxiety, and demonstrating empathic responses.

Though the interpersonal relationship with the physician begins to take shape as the patient enters the office, the nonverbal behavior of the doctor during the course of the interview will affect whether initial rapport is maintained. For example, do you find yourself preoccupied with flipping through charts or notes? To what extent are you aware of uncertainty expressed in a patient's eyes or expressions of pain? Unless you attend to what the patient is "telling" you with your eyes (as well as ears) and signal a visible readiness to listen, you are not only tuning out an important source of data, but perhaps communicating that you are disinterested in what is being said. How do you think your patients would describe your demeanor—caring, impassive, rushed, or pre-occupied? Although you may be unaware of what you are conveying, your facial expressions and body postures inadvertently tell patients a great deal about you.

Creating an atmosphere in which the patient can freely discuss circumstances and feelings related to illness is another element of rapport. Most importantly, patients should not be made fearful of negative judgments from the physician. Such fears may result in a patient hiding or misrepresenting essential information. Patients often may be reluctant to describe sexual practices, alcohol and drug use, eating habits, emotional stress, or other issues about which patients perceive the practitioner as having values quite different from their own. When approaching such topics, it is important for you to ensure confidentiality, acknowledge the potential difficulty in the discussion, and stress the relevance of an honest account for the purposes of problem solving. Once patients have opened up to you, it is imperative that you accept what they tell you in a nonjudgmental manner, even if you personally disapprove.

Because of the great number of patients seen daily, it is easy to forget the degree of concern each patient brings into the office. A conscious effort to allay anxiety is an important aspect of maintaining rapport. Be aware, for instance, of your off-hand comments that could take on fearful proportions for the patients. For example, during a pelvic examination, a gynecologist remarked to a young adolescent that he could not feel her ovaries. The girl did not respond aloud, but was left wondering if her organs had escaped to some other part of her body and what that would mean in terms of having babies. In a second instance, a family practitioner who was examining the ears of a four-year-old girl exclaimed, "That's a big red drum. This one's even worse." No further explanation was provided. Imagine the feelings this comment could engender in the child and her accompanying parent!

The physical examination deserves special attention as a situation for maintaining rapport. In one sense it has a magical quality to it. It is a time of "laying on of hands," a traditional act of healing that long precedes the practices of modern medicine. However, the physical examination frequently increases a patient's tension because so little verbal communication usually occurs. For the physician, the physical examination is a major opportunity for data gathering, but it also can and should be a time for you to give feedback to the patient. In order to provide a sense of structure and transition in this phase, you should comment briefly to the patient on what you have just seen, felt, or heard, especially if the news is reassuring. Troublesome or complicated findings, of course, need amplification and should be discussed in detail following the examination. Consider combining the review of systems with the physical examination, thus saving time and smoothly integrating a portion of verbal data gathering with the physical. A continual flow of information from you to the patient at this point in the visit anticipates basic patient anxieties and enhances the relationship you have been working to establish.

Bringing Closure

Often, the last few minutes of the interview are treated perfunctorily, which is unfortunate since the conclusion of a physician-patient encounter is likely to be what the patient remembers most. Ending the encounter should involve a summary of the problem as you see it. Furthermore, patients should be encouraged to articulate their thoughts. At least one study (Starfield, Steinwachs, Morris, Bause, Siebert & Westin 1979) indicates that problems identified by both doctor and patient as needing follow-up are more likely to be reviewed in the next visit than those mentioned only by one or the other participant. The researchers suggest several alternative solutions:

- Doctor and patient can both list important problems for the purpose of discussing and arriving at a consensus of expectations. Admittedly, this could be time-consuming.
- The patient's list can be routinely provided to the doctor at the next visit. The physician should indicate which items have been resolved, which need more attention, and which cannot be addressed.
- Patients can keep copies of a joint problem list, along with

regimens and therapies for each item. This method encourages the patient to be responsible for noting problem status at specific times so that the physician can better determine the impact of medical management.

Once problems have been jointly reviewed, subsequent steps needed to be taken following the office visit should be described. These steps might include referral to specialists or other resources, prescription of medications and instructions on their use, and an orientation toward preventive practices, all of which require clear, ample explanations. Budget time during the interview so that at the end you can discuss reasons for your directions, possible side effects or complications that might ensue from prescribed medication, and what patients can do to help themselves after they leave your office. Some patients, even when seriously ill, will be reluctant to call a physician unless they are assured that it is all right to do so and are given clear instructions on how they can contact you. Others will use no discretion and call for the slightest reasons. In either case, it is beneficial to set guidelines on this issue. Fletcher (1973) suggests that one way of increasing comprehension and subsequent follow-through is to ask the patient before leaving the office to write down the instructions you have given. Butt (1977) argues that an even more effective method is to provide patients with audiotape recordings, as well as written records, of the summary discussion.

The close of the interview can be used to engage patients actively in the choice of alternative treatments or procedures. Which path is the patient most likely to comply with, given lifestyle, belief system, and past experiences? It must be emphasized that while you may feel the conversation has ended, the anxious patient may be holding back the most troublesome question or piece of information until the last possible minute. Occasionally, the most significant patient disclosures are the last items shared. Provide the patient with a final opportunity to add to the interview. The following questions can help you check a patient's understanding of what has transpired during the interview, and encourage the verbalization of unspoken concerns.

Do you understand how we are going to deal with this problem?
Have I answered all your questions?
Are you still worried about anything we haven't discussed?

If patients raise concerns that you do not wish to address because they are not amenable to therapy or for some other reason, explain your reasons for not responding so that patients do not leave your office with unrealistic expectations or with feelings of being ignored.

The effective conclusion of an interview is more than politely ushering a patient out of the office. Instruction, influence, negotiation, and even data gathering may continue throughout this phase.

PERSUASION AND HEALING: FOLLOW-UP AND MANAGEMENT IN THE AMBULATORY SETTING

In any interpersonal endeavor it is a mistake to assume that simply telling someone what to do gives sufficient impetus for that person to follow through on the plan. Frank (1961) has written extensively on the thesis that those whose business it is to heal—medical practitioner, psychotherapist, faith healer, witch doctor—are involved in an essentially persuasive campaign to convince the patient to cooperate with them. In the same vein, Senior and Smith (1973) note that the medical curriculum omits any mention of the subject of motivating patients, a factor they feel is as crucial to successful treatment as precise diagnosis and appropriately prescribed therapy.

A few basic communication precepts can help increase patient motivation. You should become sensitive to the patient's readiness to listen to what you have to say. Receptivity is probably a combination of the patient's mood, intelligence, and immediate life circumstances, as well as the complexity and severity of the content of your message. A patient whom you judge as less ready to hear you may require that you use stylized redundancy, that is, repeating your primary message in a variety of ways throughout the conversation. Situational factors must also be considered. Too often, patients are asked to phone the physician to receive information about laboratory findings. While this medium of communication may suffice for letting someone know whether the results of a test for mononucleosis are positive, it is an inappropriate way to transmit explanations that may require visualization, as with X rays, ultrasounds, CAT scans, or information with potentially more far-reaching consequences, such as results of biopsies or fertility and pregnancy tests. Gauging an individual's readiness to receive your information requires you to pay close attention to the patient's verbal and nonverbal behaviors and requires you to adapt to the situation by determining how much time, repetition, or preliminary discussion will be needed.

Because we are focusing on interactions premised on the adult-adult relationship model, it is acceptable to think of patients being convinced rather than ordered to follow a particular management plan. One prerequisite to persuasion is for the patient to realize and acknowledge the importance of the problem at hand. Thus, your explanation must include a depiction of the disease or potential condition, anatomically, physiologically, and in terms of how it may influence the patient's way of life. The patient diagnosed with sarcoid is in need of more than a theoretical description of etiology, symptoms, and prognosis. How the progressive course of the illness may impact the patient in the context of work, recreation, and family relations will personalize and vivify your explanation and the patient's understanding of the problem.

In the case of sarcoid, for example, treatment with steroids may well complicate the patient's usual activities. Thus, treatment modes must be clearly discussed with the patient. An important aspect of persuasion is that you are able to point out that the advantages of the therapy outweigh its disadvantages, particularly in comparison with the original medical problem. With some of the most common chronic health problems—such as obesity, smoking, alcohol and drug abuse—techniques of behavior modification and support groups have proven more effective than conventionally prescribed medical regimens. These treatment modes rely heavily on immediate experience. Current experiences affecting the chronically ill patient's life appear to influence motivation to change habits or participate in therapy more than hypothetical prognostications of what will occur if the patient refuses or neglects the suggested form of treatment. At the Ochsner Clinic in New Orleans, for example, heavy smokers are ordered to return home and refrain from talking for several hours or to close off one nostril and the mouth and breathe in this fashion for several minutes, thus simulating in a graphic and meaningful way effects of cancer of the larynx or emphysema.

In cases in which the goal is to increase or decrease a behavior, such as with exercising or dieting, "the simple act of monitoring one's own . . . behavior has been shown to change the frequency of performance of that behavior" (Baranowski, Nader, Dunn & Vanderpool 1982). It stands to reason, of course, that patients are more likely to follow through on a treatment plan in which they feel they have some "ownership" or to which they have contributed. Thus, when there are viable alternatives to consider regarding type of treatment, medication, or regimen, the patient should be consulted for an opinion, if not the final decision.

Making your explanations to patients vivid and clear is an important persuasive strategy that is often overlooked by the busy practitioner. Use of examples, analogies, visual aids, and appropriate humor are all helpful techniques for reinforcing a message to a patient. Simple statistics may be used if stated in a meaningful way; to tell a mother that her baby's weight is in the seventy-fifth percentile may signify little to her unless she understands the statement to mean that of a hundred infants, only twenty-five would exceed the weight of her child. Finally, restating and emphasizing key ideas while concluding the interview are subtle but important ways of influencing and motivating the patient.

HIGH ANXIETY: TAKING A SEXUAL HISTORY

The sexual history is singled out here as a special case of data gathering because so many physicians feel uncomfortable when taking it, and the information is often omitted. The result of such neglect was vividly brought to light in an outpatient clinic recently. A thirty-year-old woman who had come in for a first visit with an entirely unrelated complaint happened to indicate on the written patient profile that she suffered severe pain during intercourse. The resident who saw her decided to follow up on this chance piece of information. The woman, married for nine years, had put aside hopes of having children and very rarely had sexual relations with her husband because of the unpleasantness associated with the experience. In the pelvic examination that followed the history, the resident was able to determine that the patient's hymen had never been completely perforated! The patient was extremely relieved to hear that her long-suffered problem could be altered and probably solved. What is remarkable and sad is that the matter had never been recognized by other practitioners she had seen.

Why is it easier to discuss bowel movements with patients than their sex lives? Both are considered taboo subjects under normal, social conditions. The difference is that in the health care context, bowel movements are more in the realm of the physiological and can be considered a symptom apart from the person. Sexual habits, however, are very much in the psychosocial realm and are an integral facet of the individual. Therefore, asking such questions feels intrusive and potentially embarrassing to many doctors.

Naturally, patients bring their own inhibitions to the situation—fears that they will be judged as abnormal, immoral, or inept if they share the secret details of body and bedroom. These are all impelling reasons for the physician to exert leadership in guiding the patient through this sort of conversation.

Perhaps the most important message for you to convey to the patient is that sex is an appropriate and acceptable topic to discuss with you. One way to communicate this to the patient more comfortably is to include the sexual history as a routine and integrated part of your medical history, as opposed to treating it as an isolated topic. For instance, it can be initiated as you find out about the patient's marital status or network of significant others. For women, it may be connected to questions regarding the menstrual cycle. It can even be included as part of the urological-genital examination. Whatever your method, the sexual history should be included in a way that makes sense to you and demonstrates to the patient that it is an expected part of the data base. Your own behavior will further substantiate this feeling. Looking the patient squarely in the eye and asking direct questions without hesitating or apologizing are strategies for you to develop.

Demonstrating a nonjudgmental attitude during the sexual history is crucial. While you personally may find various sexual behaviors immoral or undesirable, the patient whose sexual history involves such practices must not be made to feel freakish or unacceptable. A technique developed by Kinsey and his associates during his pioneering survey of human sexual behavior is to ask questions that assume everyone has engaged in every type of activity. He therefore suggested that one should not ask "Do you masturbate?" but "How often do you masturbate?" (Pomeroy 1972). Used indiscriminately, however, this technique of assumption has its limitations. For instance, some patients may not like you asking how often they engage in homosexual activities because they feel as if they are being labeled as homosexuals. Though the strategies may vary, the goal is to give the patient freedom to discuss sexual issues in a nonjudgmental climate. It is also unnecessary to ask why certain actions have been taken; this kind of question puts patients on the defensive. Your data base is more concerned with the descriptive elements of what, how, and when. Occasionally, however, you may wish to find out why the patient claims to feel a certain way in reference to portions of the sexual history.

Language use can be an unusually sensitive element during this phase of the interview because of the connotative impact of words that denote sexual anatomy and processes. This sensitivity is often heightened when the practitioner is of a different gender than the patient. Patients should be allowed to make explanations in their own choice of language, which may include vernacular and idioms. In one observed interview, for example, a college-age patient reported feeling a burning sensation from "my balls to my asshole." You must make sure that you understand idiomatic terminology and how it reflects what the patient is attempting to describe. When the words become excessively vague ("I've done petting with my boyfriend" or "I've got a sharp pain down there"), you need to encourage the patient to give a more detailed description or, in anatomical issues, even ask the patient to point to the area in question. For your part, you should use language that you are comfortable with, providing the patient can understand you; physicians sometimes resort to inappropriately technical terms as a way of covering their own embarrassment. You should not use euphemisms or feel compelled to use the patient's choice of language if it is unfamiliar to you. Such attempts usually come off as false and stilted.

During this or any other part of the interview, you may need to explore further. You should probe topics in which the patient shows particular interest or signs of concerns. Be aware of behavioral inconsistencies. If the patient claims that sexual relations with his or her spouse are "okay," but looks tense or distracted, further attempts to question are in order.

A standard interviewing strategy to reduce tension is to begin with general, nonthreatening questions and then proceed to the more specific ones. Wiens and Brazman (1977) suggest for the sexual history openers such as, "Have there been any changes in your sexual feelings or behavior?" or "How satisfying is your sexual life?" More detailed follow-up probes might include "How often do you have intercourse?" "Do you mean you feel disappointed with yourself, your partner, or both?" "Do you mean you sometimes lose your erection when you don't want to?" or "Is your erection sufficient to continue with intercourse?" If a subject comes up about which the patient is extremely embarrassed or reticent, let it drop for the moment, but try to approach it again since the patient's aversion probably indicates that something significant is afoot.

Communicating about sexual practices and problems as a regular part of taking the history allows patients to feel accepted, to bring to light questions and symptoms that they have been afraid to discuss with anyone else, to gain needed information, and to be referred to knowledgeable sources, if necessary.

MEDICAL INTERVIEW SELF-ASSESSMENT CHECKLIST

Completing a medical interview self-assessment checklist (Foley & Sharf 1981) can help you identify and further develop the communication skills that you use during the medical interview. Recent evidence indicates that patient assessment behaviors can be considerably sharpened and enriched through increased awareness and practice with an itemized checklist (Stillman, May, Meyer, Rutala, Veach & Montgomery 1981). Therefore, the checklist in Figure 3.3, which summarizes the communication skills discussed in this chapter, is to be used as a self-assessment tool to review physician-patient interaction in your own practice.

The checklist can be used with audiotape or videotape. In either case, of course, the patient's permission should be obtained in advance. Audiotaping an interview can provide you with useful feedback about the rate at which you interview, the kinds of questions you ask, and the proportion of time spent on various portions of the interview.

Videotape is the far more powerful tool for self-assessment (Cassata & Clements 1978). Although it has been used increasingly in medical student education, it is rarely employed among physicians in practice. If you have access to videotape facilities as most hospitals do, be sure the camera is focused on both you and the patient. Play back the tape without sound to gain a picture of your nonverbal behaviors on the checklist. Play it a second time with sound and make note of the other items that could be improved. Schedule a second videotape a few weeks later and again review it with the checklist to see whether the desired shifts have taken place. The time spent will be well worth it.

FIGURE 3.3   *Medical Interview Self-Assessment Checklist*

	Not done	Only partially or rarely done	Completely or usually done	Not applicable
Beginning the interview				
Putting the patient at ease				
Initiates a visit that puts the patient at ease				
Shows respect for patient by attending to needs for privacy and comfort				
During the interview				
Eliciting information				
Uses open-ended questions to facilitate patient responses when appropriate				
Allows patient opportunity to explain story in own words without unnecessary interruptions				
Offers possible responses when patient appears unable to answer				
Rephrases or repeats questions if needed to enhance understanding				
Clarifies areas of confusion or inconsistencies				
Inquires how well patient understands present illness				
Uses language appropriate to patient's age and background				
Uses additional forms of communication (diagrams, written materials, x-rays, EEGs, etc.)				
Avoids verbal habits (continual okays, uh-huhs, nodding) that may be misunderstood by patient				
Maintaining direction				
Paces the interview comfortably and efficiently				
Uses periodic summaries				
Makes clear transitions from one step of the interview to another				
Interrupts unnecessary patient rambling to maintain focus				
Uses pauses to encourage patient response				

FIGURE 3.3 Medical Interview Self-Assessment Checklist (Cont'd)

	Not done	Only partially or rarely done	Completely or usually done	Not applicable
Maintaining rapport				
Maintains eye contact				
Uses nonverbal communication (office seating arrangement, use of charts, posture, facial expressions, touch) appropriately				
Allows opportunities for patient to express feelings about current illness and other issues				
Accepts patient's values in a nonjudgmental manner				
Remains sensitive to language or behavior that might arouse patient anxiety				
Explains the need for requesting certain data in order to reduce patient anxiety				
Deals with patient's questions and concerns				
Deals with patient's nonverbally communicated concerns				
Reinforces and encourages patient's abilities to cope				
Ending the interview:				
Bringing closure				
Informs patient about next steps when appropriate				
Allows patient opportunity to ask additional questions or add to the interview				
Negotiates differences in physician and patient thinking until consensus is achieved				
Provides closing statements that facilitate a comfortable ending				

SUMMARY

Chapter 3 has advocated the adult-adult model of physician-patient communication as most appropriate for ambulatory settings. In the management of chronic illness and health care prevention in the outpatient milieu, the patient must assume major responsibility and should collaborate as fully as possible with the physician in the formulation of diagnosis, treatment plan, and follow-up.

The outpatient environment itself can be arranged in ways to create a positive impression and facilitate interaction. The face-to-face encounter between doctor and patient is discussed in terms of five communicative functions of the practitioner: putting the patient at ease, eliciting information, maintaining direction, maintaining rapport, and bringing closure. Allaying patient anxiety, identifying patient perceptions, and negotiating differences in thinking between physician and patient are guidelines that should be kept in mind throughout a medical interview.

Physician-patient communication has a decidedly persuasive aspect that entails being sensitive to a patient's readiness to receive information, as well as clear, vivid, and emphatic explanations. Sexual history taking is treated as a particular communication problem for many practitioners with specific suggestions for improving results.

Chapter 4 will now build upon the principles of physician-patient communication presented thus far, while exploring the special circumstances of the hospitalized patient.

References

Baranowski, T., Nader, P. R., Dunn, K., & Vanderpool, N. A. Family self-help: promoting changes in health behavior. *Journal of Communication,* 1982, *32,* 161–72.

Butt, H. R. A method for better physician-patient communication. *Annals of Internal Medicine,* 1977, *86,* 478–80.

Cassata, D. M., & Clements, P. W. Teaching communication skills through videotape feedback: A rural health program. *Biosciences Communications,* 1978, *4,* 39–50.

Fletcher, C. M. *Communication in medicine.* Abingdon, Great Britain: The Nuffield Provincial Hospitals Trust, 1973.

Foley, R., & Sharf, B. F. The five interviewing techniques most frequently overlooked by primary care physicians. *Behavioral Medicine,* 1981, *8,* 26–31.

Frank, J. D. *Persuasion and healing: A comparative study of psychotherapy.* Baltimore: The Johns Hopkins Press, 1961.

Pendleton, D. Personal communication, May 5, 1982.

Pomeroy, W. B. *Dr. Kinsey and the Institute for Sex Research*. New York: Harper & Row, 1972.

Senior, B., & Smith, B. A. The motivation of the patient as a neglected factor in therapy. *Journal of Medical Education*, 1973, *48*, 589–91.

Starfield, B., Steinwachs, D., Morris, I., Bause, G., Siebert, S., & Westin, C. Patient-doctor agreement about problems needing follow-up visit. *Journal of the American Medical Association*, 1979, *242*, 344–46.

Stillman, P. L., May, J. R., Meyer, D. M., Rutala, P. J., Veach, T. L., & Montgomery, A. B. A collaborative effort to study methods of teaching physical examination skills. *Journal of Medical Education*, 1981, *56*, 301–6.

Stoeckle, J. D., & Barsky, A. J. Attributions: Uses of social science knowledge in the "doctoring" of primary care. In L. Eisenberg and A. Kleinman (Eds.), *The relevance of social science for medicine*. Boston: D. Reidel Publishing Co., 1980.

Szasz, T. S., & Hollender, M. H. A contribution to the philosophy of medicine. *Archives of Internal Medicine*, 1956, *97*, 585–92.

Weins, A., & Brazman, R. A rationale and method for the sexual history in family practice. *Journal of Family Practice*, 1977, *5*, 213–15.

Communicating with the Hospitalized Patient

The last few moments of consciousness before the effect of anesthesia for surgery begins epitomize the situation of the hospitalized patient. Will I wake up again? If I do wake up, will I feel sicker than I do now before surgery? What parts of my body will be gone after the surgery? At this time, the patient gives up all control and self-determination to the team of physicians in charge; like it or not, the patient must permit the relationship to become one of ultimate submission. Although the experience of every person who is hospitalized is not always this dramatic, the same themes generally characterize dynamics between doctors and patients in hospitals, varying only in degree of intensity.

Chapter 3 emphasized the opportunity for choice and personal responsibility as an essential aspect of care for the ambulatory patient that should be taken into account by the administering physician. The hospitalized patient, like the traveler in a foreign land described earlier, experiences unfamiliar sounds, smells, and tastes. Suddenly the hospitalized patient has an overwhelming sense of powerlessness and lack of autonomy. Uncertainties about the nature of illness or outcome of treatment are intensified by the sense of other people being in charge. Mundane activities, such as bathing, eating, and elimination, are often regulated and monitored by external agents known as members of the health care team. Normal patterns of modesty and privacy are violated. Unidentified strangers in white coats may ask questions with answers never before disclosed, and view parts of a patient's anatomy heretofore not seen even by members of that individual's own family.

At the steep cost of at least several hundred dollars a day, the hospitalized patient finds that the outer shell of the body, which usually serves as a buffer from the outside world, is open to all sorts of invasions and interventions. At the very least, the body is exposed, touched, probed, and examined. Needles, tubes, X rays, enemas, as well as scalpels are tools of the medical profession that give or take fluids, leave deposits, scars, and sometimes pain. Without the protection of its outside armor, the psyche of a patient may have to adapt considerably in order to protect itself against the onslaught of medical assistance.

Finally, there is an aspect of modern hospitalization that transcends the risks of human interaction. Technology. Ultrasounds, CAT scans, fetal and cardiac monitors, electroencephalograms, and echocardiograms are relatively new forms of medical technology that further impede establishing human relationships. From the patient's vantage point, the machinery adds to feelings of bewilderment, impotency, and depersonalization in this strange environment. The diagnostic or therapeutic benefits of technology can be extraordinary, but their impact on patients should not be overlooked.

All of this is not new to you, of course. You may see the inside of a hospital almost every day. However, within its very familiarity lies the danger to physician-patient relationships. The corridors, uniforms, and equipment that have become second nature to you are worrisome and strange to patients. What seems a moment to you on a hurried schedule of rounds may be an unbearably long period to the confined or pain-ridden individual. Your very comings and goings become objects of patients' scrutiny. It is easy for you to overlook how such milieu and sensations can affect the patient. Good communication cannot be a panacea for the discomforts and fears that beset the hospitalized patient, but it can help alleviate some, and perhaps compensate for others.

ACUTE ILLNESS

Acute episodes of illness are usually responsible for changing the status of a patient from ambulatory to hospitalized; sometimes, of course, signs of disease, such as a suspicious lump, precede actual feelings of illness. Severe bouts of sickness alter the resources of an individual and, necessarily, the doctor-patient relationship. Perhaps most strikingly, acute illness renders patients particularly dependent on their physicians. Szasz and Hollender (1956) describe such relationships in developmental terms, in contrast with the adult-adult relationship presented in Chapter 3 as appropriate to the chronically ill, ambulatory patient.

Parent-Infant Relationships

In some situations, the patient's medical condition dictates almost total dependence on the physician and other health professionals, with no opportunity for the patient to participate in the treatment process. Szasz and Hollender cite examples such as patients who are comatose, in intensive care, or brought into the emergency room in states of trauma or other crises. The metaphor for this type of relationship is parent-infant. The physician must act upon, do something to the patient, a la the traditional medical model; communication is therefore one-way, and lacks feedback or any type of verbal interaction. While this is not a preferred communicative mode when other choices are available, in these circumstances it is clearly the most appropriate. As with the parent-infant prototype, decision making is done on behalf of, but not by, the patient. Also, as with preverbal infants, many patients in crisis, even those who are only semiconscious, are likely to perceive and respond to attempts at nonverbal communication, particularly touch.

Parent-Child Relationships

Most hospitalized patients are not totally passive and are capable of varying degrees of interaction with their physicians and other health professionals. Their resources for contributing to their own health care will depend in part on the nature and extent of both their illness and treatment procedures. However, by virtue of hospitalization, patients automatically assume a socially created status which sociologist Talcott Parsons (1951) has characterized classically as the "sick role." While participating in the sick role, individuals are exempt from performance of normal social obligations and from the responsibility of their own debilitated conditions. Simultaneously, those recognized as sick are obligated to seek technically competent help, to be motivated to get well, and to trust the doctor or, put in other words, to accept an inferior position in an asymmetrical relationship. Clearly, Parsons has depicted a relationship of dependence, much as a child depends on a parent. There may be differential amounts of dependence; a toddler is necessarily more reliant than a teenager, but neither is capable of adult independence and autonomy. Ambulatory patients are sometimes imbued with the characteristics of the sick role for periods of time, but it is more difficult to maintain consistently outside an institutionalized setting.

The communication that accompanies the parent-child relationship can be described as advisory-compliant (which Szasz and Hollender describe as guidance-cooperation). In the advisory capacity, the physician assumes an authoritative, leadership role in terms of defining the patient's medical situation and giving orders for treatment. The patient is an active participant in the communication with the complementary role of accepting the doctor's definition and complying with orders. Like an obedient child, the patient is expected to follow through on the doctor's advice, even when the consequences are distasteful, with the assumption that the physician "knows best" and that the decision is for the patient's "own good." The patient is not expected to argue, question, or disagree. Szasz and Hollender point out that this relationship format is appropriate when patients are suffering from acute illnesses, such as persons recovering from myocardial infarction or meningitis. Because this parent-child type of interaction is marked by the patient's dependence on the medical practitioner, one of the aspects of the relationship most reassuring to the patient is the doctor's accessibility. Communication with even the most compliant of patients is enhanced by providing them with information, support, and, more fundamentally, evidence of the physician's involvement through his or her presence. One patient we know who was hospitalized for surgery became increasingly irritated after repeated requests to talk with his surgeon were ignored. As a last resort, he sent a telegram to the doctor emphasizing his urgent need to speak with him. The surgeon appeared in the patient's room within a half hour of receiving the telegram. Certainly, this was an ingenious move on the part of the patient, but should such strategies be necessary?

As the patient's illness progresses from an acute to a chronic stage or from sickness to health, the mode of communication should change accordingly, from the parent-child toward the adult-adult level of functioning. With situational modifications and adaptations, most of the advice offered in Chapter 3 for improving communication with patients is also applicable to the hospitalized patient. Further considerations are necessary to cope with the problems and peculiarities specific to hospital milieu.

BEDSIDE MANNER

"Bedside manner" may be old-fashioned terminology, but its importance to the physician-patient relationship has not decreased over the years. The most basic aspect of establishing rapport with the hospitalized patient is *personalizing the encounter*. Making introductions is an obvious, but often neglected, way to start. During a stay at a modern, particularly a teaching, hospital, an individual is apt to be seen by a cadre of health practitioners, many of whose functions are unknown or mistakenly supposed by the patient. Doctors are probably the most confusing lot, by virtue of their number, variety, and the scant amount of time actually spent with the patient. Without a scorecard, a patient can have difficulty knowing a fourth-year medical student from an attending physician, a fellow in cardiology from a resident in surgery. Consider the perspective of one patient who was observed as he experienced his first hospitalization. He had been admitted at night and the next morning was amazed to see his assigned physician march into his room accompanied by eleven other staff and students. When the doctor had finished his examination and was about to leave, the patient called him over and asked in a worried tone, "Am I *that* sick?" referring to all the people who had come to see him. "We don't know," his physician curtly replied. "Why were all these people here?" the patient continued to wonder. "They were observing," the doctor answered. Offering no elaboration, the physician exited. The patient was left with an expression of anxious concern on his face.

Given the complex milieu of a hospital service, one suggestion is to actually provide the patient with a "scorecard," that is, a printed list showing photographs of the staff assigned to the service with a brief written description of the function of each staff member. If that idea seems extreme to you, put yourself in the place of a patient hospitalized for a gastrointestinal problem. Conceivably, this person could be seen by an attending physician, a junior attending, a fellow, one or more residents, one or more medical students, several nurses, a social worker, an X-ray technician, and a dietician! On an individual basis, it is incumbent upon you to take the initiative in addressing patients by name, introducing yourself by name, and clarifying your function in the case. In the context of a teaching hospital, you should explain to your patients from the outset (or as soon as they are well enough to converse) the necessity for the presence of learners or ancillary staff. Furthermore, whenever you enter a patient's room with other people in tow, make reference to who they are and what they are doing there; for example, "This is Dr. O'Brien from the Rheumatology section, whom I've asked to consult on your case; he will help me examine your leg today" or "The young people in this group are third-year medical students who are here to observe today so they can learn about your problem."

During rounds many clinicians can be seen standing at each patient's bedside seeming poised to travel on to the next stop. Even if one is not in a hurry, the stance suggests impatience and inhibits patients from feeling free to say what is on their minds. Pulling up a chair next to the bed does not require you to stay longer than you wish, but the seated position allows you to have level eye contact with your patients and is a more convincing indication that you are being attentive to what they have to say.

Good listening does require that you clear your mind from other thoughts long enough to be open to what the patient is now saying and doing, as well as a sincere desire on your part to hear what is being said. In other words, being a good listener while on rounds is no different than exercising the same skill in other situations; listening requires involvement with the other person and the specific circumstances in which communication is taking place. It is not hard to understand why patients often mistake a medical student for the attending doctor or admit that they wish the medical student were in charge of their case. Many rarely see their assigned physicians. When they do, there is limited opportunity for interchange to take place, whereas medical students are more available to them. In one instance, a forty-seven-year-old woman had been admitted to the hospital for open heart surgery on her mitral valve. Since this patient had been worked up extensively by residents and attending staff during a previous admission for cardiac catheterization, she had not been examined in depth on the day of her current admission. However, a fourth-year medical student did come to her room to do a history and physical and talked with the patient for an hour and a half. She expressed to him her worries about her family and the outcome of the operation. She also asked him when the surgery would be performed. He replied the time would be decided when the chief of cardiology made rounds. The following day, the chief of cardiology arrived for rounds with an entourage of a dozen people, including the medical student bringing up the rear. The section chief told the patient she was ready for surgery, which would be scheduled for the next day. The patient answered, "Fine, but I'll have to wait until I discuss this with *my* doctor." "And who is your doctor?" roared the chief, annoyed that his judgment might be questioned. "Why, Dr. Foster," said the patient, pointing to the embarrassed medical student.

The concept of personalization is interrelated with the theme of *dignifying the individual patient.* The plight of the hospitalized patient is one in which the decorum of everyday life is stripped away. Perhaps the most obvious illustration is the pajamas or dressing gown that is the uniform of a patient; patients must sometimes encounter their professionally attired physicians clad only in bedsheets. Often they are prevented from behaving in characteristic ways or performing routine activities by pain, disabling ailments, or fatigue; if disease has not limited their capacities, treatment modes or medications frequently do. It is all the more important for doctors not to contribute to further degradation or regression while interacting with acutely ill patients. When confronted with renal failure in a patient, you must as a medical problem solver compare the characteristics of this case with similar instances of renal failure that you have treated or about which you have read. However, when visiting the patient it is equally necessary to acknowledge that individual's experience of the problem and to recognize his or her unique limitations and resources in dealing with it. Only in this way can you communicate to patients that they are not being viewed as diseased organs or clinical specimens. Patients should also be encouraged to maintain their own sense of self and personality by perhaps keeping some personal effects, jewelry, a bed jacket, glasses, or cosmetics by the bed to help them feel distinct in the midst of pervasive institutionalization. By taking account of the patient's individuality, you not only contribute to preserving a sense of personal dignity, but also help move the physician-patient relationship from a parent-child stance toward an adult-adult mode of functioning.

The activities of hospitalized medical care impinge greatly on normal expectations of privacy. In few other situations could personal talks with family or friends be disrupted at any time simply for the purpose of carrying out a technical procedure, such as drawing blood. In no other place would an individual be required to update reports on patterns of flatulence or excretion. In short, maintenance of privacy is not a prime objective in the design of hospital activities, nor should it necessarily be. The medical practitioner should, however, keep in mind that the delicate situations that occur in hospitals require creating a sense of privacy for the patient when it does not naturally exist.

Imagine yourself in the following scene. A Code Blue alert is sounded on a general medicine service signifying that a patient has suffered cardiac arrest. Medical and nursing staff from all over the floor come running to the designated room, along with all medical, nursing, and pharmacy students in the area, as well as a few "official" but nonmedical hospital personnel who happen to be there at the time. Almost thirty people have crowded into the patient's room or are gathered in the hallway to watch from the door. The curtain is never drawn around the ailing patient's bed nor is the other patient sharing the room wheeled out until the crisis passes. The twenty-six individuals who are observing rather than actively participating in the emergency care are asked to stand back, but are never asked to leave. In the meantime, the sister of the critically ill patient has come up to the floor and is making her way to the room. By a stroke of luck, a nurse recognizes her and ushers her off to the waiting room before she reaches her destination. Despite continuous efforts, the patient cannot be resuscitated. The phone by her bed rings and is answered by a nurse who says, "I'm sorry, she's not here." Hanging up the phone, the nurse giggles to another, "She's *really* not here!" After fifteen minutes have elapsed, a nurse inside the room closes the door, saying to the observers huddled outside, "There's been enough gawking here." The other patient takes in the whole scene in horror and confusion.

This is a description of an actual, not a fictitious, event. Perhaps you have been part of similar ones. The issue is not the treatment given by the medical staff, but the quality of care that permits one patient to die in a public, undignified manner and forces another patient to be an unwilling observer.

In general, physician-patient relationships will be enhanced to the degree the patient feels a sense of dignity and the comfort of privacy. The bedside curtain should be drawn regularly when you come to talk and examine patients. Even if the room is not shared, the curtain is protection against the interruption of other staff and visitors to the room. It may be necessary at times to clear the room of other people or, if circumstances allow, to talk with the patient in another setting. We recently watched an attending orthopedic surgeon break in on two medical students collecting a history from his patient. In front of all of us, he asked hurriedly, "Mr. Rodriguez, do you have any questions about your surgery tomorrow?" The patient asked one question, then declined to ask further. For his part, the attending physician encouraged no other inquiries and left quickly. After the doctor had gone, the patient expressed to the two students, whom he had met only a half hour before, many fears he had about the risks of the surgery and admitted that he did not understand many aspects of the procedure. Unfortunately, the manner and setting in which the orthopedist asked whether the patient had questions communicated that this was only a perfunctory exercise and discouraged the patient from speaking his mind. Privacy helps physicians as well as patients express themselves. You should not feel intrusive asking visitors to step out for a few minutes or requesting that the patient turn off the television or radio in order to facilitate conversation.

GIVING INFORMATION

In treating the ambulatory patient, the doctor gathers much information through interviewing, but also supplies the patient with information while explaining medical problems, providing directions for self-management, and encouraging preventive measures. Communicating information has perhaps even greater consequences when talking with the hospitalized patient because of the complexity of the hospital setting and the dependence of the acutely ill patient on the practitioner.

There are many subjects to discuss and explain before and during a patient's hospitalization. First is the *nature of the disease or medical problem* itself. Even when a patient is admitted for observation and diagnostic testing, an understanding of the range of possibilities at least helps define the situation for the patient and his or her significant others who are otherwise anxious about the unknown. Well-intentioned clinicians sometimes underestimate both the ability and willingness of patients to comprehend the illness at hand. This tendency is illustrated in an interaction that occurred between a pediatric neurologist and the parents of a three-year-old patient who showed signs of muscle weakness. After completing a history and physical diagnosis, the physician told the parents that blood tests and an electromyography would need to be done. Since he made no mention of diagnosis, the mother asked what he thought the problem could be. "Well, it's either congenital myopathy or myasthenias gravis," he answered, making no attempt to explain either condition. The mother then requested that he write down the two terms, to which the doctor replied, "That's not necessary. You'll only want to look up those words and you'll worry yourself." It seems incredible that he could not or would not recognize what sorts of anxiety could result from his refusal to help identify or define the problem.

The problem, after all, does belong to the patient who must live with it. Yet it is not uncommon to find hospitalized patients who cannot tell about their sickness in their own words, other than describe symptomatology. To help alleviate this situation, it is useful for the physician to explain the etiology and course of a disease, using lay language and simple diagrams that depict internal anatomy, which is often unknown to the patient.

Second, *explain diagnostic and treatment procedures.* Without an adequate understanding of events happening to them and occurring around them, patients will construe their own interpretations and could be unnecessarily alarmed. One patient was admitted at night with, among other symptoms, a hoarse cough. Because the man's history indicated a previous hospitalization for tuberculosis, his hospital room was marked "contagious" and all people who entered had to wear a mask. Not surprisingly, the patient assumed he had tuberculosis, though tuberculin tests performed the following day proved negative. The clinical staff, of course, was correct in taking precautions until a diagnosis could be confirmed. The problem was the result of not informing the patient that the procedure was precautionary. In this case, as in many others, a simple explanation that orients the patient to present or changing circumstances will suffice.

Progressively complicated situations and procedures necessitate correspondingly detailed comments. In terms they are able to understand, patients should be told

- why a procedure is performed,
- how they can expect to feel during or following,
- when they can expect to hear results, and
- what the results are, once they are known.

Although it is often felt that giving patients this much information will cause them to worry unnecessarily, the opposite reaction is frequently the case. Knowing what is ahead can allow patients a chance to prepare psychologically for the experience. For example, anticipating that one will be bedridden or weakened for several days lets one "take care of business," finish urgent tasks and make future arrangements before entering the hospital. In the instance of the pediatric neurologist described above, the mother asked what the electromyography entails. The doctor replied that it is the neurological equivalent of an electrocardiogram, which was a familiar procedure to her. With this answer, the mother assumed the EMG would not be painful or scary for her three-year-old child. When she found out from other sources what the test involved, she felt deceived, very distrustful, and severed the relationship with the neurologist. She later sought a second opinion and eventually allowed the procedure to be done, but only after she was able to talk extensively with her daughter about the upcoming event. Shaping the patient's expectations also can prevent subsequent alarm, as with the myomectomy patient who has been told she may have some bleeding during recuperation.

An additional reason for emphasizing the importance of information-giving skills in the hospital is the high incidence of organic mental disorders in hospitalized patients. These reactions, usually transient, occur in 5 to 15 percent of hospitalized patients, particularly in the elderly and those receiving many drugs simultaneously. While organic factors (for example, hypoxia, drug side effects, and hypoglycemia) are usually the precipitating agents, the interpersonal environment of the hospital plays a critical role in predisposing the patient to such a problem. Clear, precise, and continual communication between the patient and health care team is highly desirable as a way of combating patient disorientation and psychological distress.

Perhaps, the most critical occasion in making explanations to the hospitalized patient or to one who is about to be hospitalized is when a decision must be made—whether to have a cardiac bypass, whether to have a lumpectomy or mastectomy, whether local or general anesthesia will be used. In theory, informed consent should ensure that pros and cons of both the proposed treatment and existing alternatives are reviewed with the patient, and that the patient is aware of potential deleterious consequences as well as benefits before making the decision. In practice, the patient is frequently presented with a document written in incomprehensible "legalese" that leads to cursory reading and inadequate recall of what was stated (Cassileth, Nukkis, Sutton-Smith & March 1980). Written consent forms that are easily understood, accompanied by a thorough oral presentation with time allotted to encourage questions is what is required for truly informed consent.

Hospitalized patients encounter a confusing array of persons supposedly responsible for their health care. In addition to the possibility of contributing to depersonalization, this factor can add to problems with the patient's decision making. The patient may not know with whom to bring up questions or fears, and thus never verbalizes them. Or, as often occurs, the patient may mistakenly assume that a concern expressed to a nurse will be transmitted automatically to a physician. Because the potential for blocking pathways for efficient communication in the hospital is high, it is important that special care be taken to avoid the more obvious or predictable difficulties. You should make sure that patients have a chance to ask you questions, and be certain that your involvement in their cases is clear enough so that they have an idea of what sort of questions would be appropriate to address to you, thereby increasing their comfort level. Naturally patients may pose queries to you that should be answered by a colleague; your responsibility then becomes one of acting as a liaison with the proper person so that the patient's question is not ignored or forgotten.

FACILITATING PATIENT SUPPORT NETWORKS

Depending on the types of problems you tend to see in your practice, it may be useful for you to adopt the role of facilitator of patient communication. The therapeutic effects of patient support groups, that is, the sharing of feelings and experiences among individuals with similar maladies, has been well documented (for example, Lieberman, Borman, et al, 1979). Although patients, volunteers, or health-oriented organizations like the American Cancer Society may initiate such groups on their own, the doctor's acknowledgment and approval of these groups can be a strong influence on patients to join. Furthermore, physicians frequently are in the position of treating two or more people with the same or similar problems, sometimes at the same stage of development. When the patient is in the hospital facing the prospects of a traumatic surgery such as a mastectomy, colostomy, or limb amputation; painful or debilitating treatment such as radiation and chemotherapy for cancer; or a radically altered lifestyle caused by diabetes, epilepsy, heart disease, strokes, and so on, talking with someone else who has experienced or is similarly facing the same circumstances can be especially beneficial.

WHEN CARE REPLACES CURE: COMMUNICATING WITH THE SEVERELY ILL AND DYING

As you know, the physician is frequently the bearer of bad tidings. Doctors are regularly called upon to discuss with their patients such issues as the need to amputate a limb, the advisability of sterilization, or the confirmation of a diagnosis of a progressively debilitating disease, such as systemic lupus erythematosus, Huntington's chorea, or multiple sclerosis. It is therefore not difficult to understand the impulses of an attending neurologist recently observed on hospital rounds. After he gave a detailed explanation of the patient's illness, confirming a diagnosis of multiple sclerosis in highly technical terms to a group of medical students, the patient asked directly, "Doctor, do I have multiple sclerosis?" "We'll have to look at further test results before we know for sure," he replied, despite the information he had just shared with the students. No one enjoys being in such an uncomfortable situation and many of us may have chosen at times to procrastinate or even hide unpleasant information.

It is always a matter of subjective judgment when to share bad news with a patient, but some patients do ask for information in a straightforward way, indicating a desire to know. While a number of people have made the case for the beneficial effects of lying to patients (De Beauvoir 1966; Lipkin 1979), we feel nondisclosure of pertinent information limits an individual's ability to make choices about the remainder of his or her life, which may include the choice of denying what has been discussed. Cousins (1982) has written eloquently of communication strategies for these difficult situations:

> Is it possible to communicate negative information in a way that is received by the patient as a challenge rather than as a death sentence? . . . Physicians . . . have developed techniques for communicating without crippling . . . . They set a stage conducive to treatment and recovery. They do not minimize the seriousness of the patient's condition. Instead, they put their emphasis on the strategy of combat. They propose a partnership. They describe what modern medical science has to offer and then describe what the patient has to offer . . . . For a patient to be told that two of every five persons with a certain illness do not last out the year is not as useful or as motivating as to be told that three of five patients overcome their illness. The basic purpose here is *not to destroy the hope* that provides an essential environment for healing. (p. 588)

Cousins also reminds us of the important influence of the physician-patient relationship; that patients "want to feel that it makes a difference to the physician, a very big difference, whether they live or die" (p. 589).

Because people often spend their final days in the hospital, perhaps the most important point is not to *avoid* communicating with the dying patient. For a variety of reasons, including the unresolved fears associated with our own deaths and our inability to overcome the patient's problem, most of us would prefer to avoid the presence of dying patients. Or, when in the presence of a dying patient, many of us become businesslike and force the conversation into tightly guarded discussions about the medical treatment. Conversely, some physicians compensate for this fear or anxiety by forcing patients into deep philosophical discussions in order to penetrate their feelings about dying. What physicians need to be aware of is the specific feelings of each patient regarding if, how, when, and with whom one feels most comfortable about discussing imminent death.

Kubler-Ross (1969) made excellent observations about the stages of death: denial, anger, depression, bargaining, and acceptance. Unfortunately, her work has led to several misconceptions by people working with dying patients. The first misconception is that every patient will become the "ideal" and pass through each step in the sequence described, which is far from the truth. There are as many ways to approach death as there are personalities in the population. Some patients continue with denial or anger, for example, from the time they are told the news until they die. It is important for the physician to respect individual differences and not expect patients to move toward an ideal acceptance of death.

A second misconception is that the physician and the health care team have a responsibility to help patients move toward accepting death. Rather, once a patient is aware of having a terminal prognosis, the physician's responsibility is to be available, to listen to the patient's concerns and feelings about death, if and when the patient desires to discuss the situation. Neither should physicians feel slighted or think that their duties are being taken away if patients select a friend, family member, spiritual advisor, medical student, or nurse with whom to discuss more intimate thoughts and feelings about death.

The physician's continuous communicative goals in relating to progressively ill and dying patients should be

- to make the patient comfortable,
- to neither raise false hopes nor deny the near universal hope that death may be thwarted,
- to be accessible without being intrusive, and
- to maintain sensitivity and empathy in talking with the patient without becoming too burdened with emotions to be of service.

SUMMARY

Chapter 4 has built upon the precepts of good physician-patient communication described in Chapter 3, with special emphasis on the effects of hospital milieu and acute illness. Lack of environmental and self-control, the ubiquity of technology, and deleterious physical and psychological consequences of illness and treatment are factors that contribute to a more dependent relationship between patient and physician. In lieu of the adult-adult model of interaction, communication with the hospitalized patient more appropriately takes the form of parent-infant or parent-child interaction. Communication skills for the physician in these circumstances center on being available, personalizing the encounter, and dignifying the individual patient. Giving information about the nature of the medical problem, treatment procedures and results, and informed consent are crucial to the patient's ability to adjust to the situation and cope with the illness. Suggested strategies for talking with critically ill and dying patients include providing information in a straightforward manner, continuing interpersonal contact during the final stages of illness, and respecting the individual's reaction to his or her condition.

Although the designated patient is the doctor's major responsibility, it is often necessary to interact with a patient's family, friends, and acquaintances. Chapter 5 will explore ways of coping with these situations.

References

Cassileth, B. R., Nukkis, R. V., Sutton-Smith, K., & March, V. Informed consent— why are its goals imperfectly realized. *New England Journal of Medicine,* 1980, *302,* 896–902.

Cousins, N. The physician as communicator. *Journal of the American Medical Association,* 1982, *248,* 587–89.

De Beauvoir, S. [*A very easy death.*] (P. O'Brien, trans). New York: G. P. Putnam's Sons, 1966.

Kubler-Ross, E. *On death and dying.* New York: MacMillan, 1969.

Lieberman, M. A., Borman, L. D., et al. *Self-help groups for coping with crisis: Origins, members, processes, and impact.* San Francisco; Jossey-Bass, 1979.

Lipkin, M. On lying to patients. *Newsweek,* June 14, 1979, 13.

Parsons, T. *The social system.* Glencoe, Illinois: The Free Press, 1951.

Szasz, T. S., & Hollender, M. H. A contribution to the philosophy of medicine. *Archives of internal medicine,* 1956, *97,* 585–92.

CHAPTER 5

Network Communication: The Patient's Family and Significant Others

A Rubik's Cube is a puzzle composed of many movable, interlocking smaller cubes of six different colors. The object of the game is to arrange the smaller cubes in such a way that each of the six sides of the larger cube will appear as a solid and distinct color. In trying to solve the puzzle, moving any one smaller cube changes the face of the whole, larger cube. Therein lies the frustration and the challenge of the game.

Families have some of the same characteristics as the Rubik's Cube. An event that occurs with one family member may well influence the behavior and health of others. *Event* is used here in a broad sense; examples of common significant events include marriage, divorce, birth, death, onset or progression of illness, recovery from illness, change in work responsibilities, and so forth. Clearly, the family unit is a likely breeding ground for allergies and infectious diseases on a purely biological basis. A lesser acknowledged fact is the connection between the psychological health of the family and physical illness. Haggerty (1968) found that common family crises, such as the death of a grandparent, change of residence, loss of the father's job, and so on occurred significantly more often in the two-week period before the appearance of a streptococcal infection in a family member than in the two weeks afterward. Haggerty hypothesized that such crises serve to lower a patient's resistance to infection. Thus, the state of healthiness or illness of one individual may be reflective or symbolic of the welfare of other people in the family.

By the same token, any change that results from your treatment of a patient may have repercussions from other family members. A typical example is the adolescent son or daughter who acts out family tensions and problems with alcoholic drinking, drug use, or anorexia nervosa. Often the teenager is presented to the family doctor or a psychiatrist as the problematic person or black sheep of the family. If the physician is able to treat the symptoms in such a way that they begin to disappear, it has been observed in numerous cases that another person in the family, formerly regarded as healthy, will show signs of illness. Similarly, your attempts to treat patients may be sabotaged by family dynamics. One family practitioner reports seeing a patient over several years who had a stream of psychosomatic complaints—headaches, chest pain, back-aches, and stomach upsets. Once one ailment had been taken care of, another one would appear. This patient was a single male adult still living at home with his parents. An older brother had died of muscular dystrophy, his father was an alcoholic, and his mother was withdrawn and depressed. His symptoms tended to flare up when the father's drinking or the mother's depression became particularly stressful. In effect he was the official symptom bearer for the family. Thus, without addressing etiology embedded in family dynamics, the physician's treatment of symptoms proved superficial and ineffective.

On the other hand, the resources of the family network may be used constructively to manage both chronic and acute illness. For many Americans conditioned by geographic mobility and social norms, the nuclear family is the unit of influence in both decision making and support giving. In some subcultures the traditional importance of the extended family has been preserved. It is not unusual, for example, to see several members of Hispanic families crowded into a patient's room, day after day. Such concerted family solidarity is often viewed by the health care team as a disturbance or nuisance, although it may be a source of psychological strength and aid to the patient. For certain patients a network of friends and colleagues may serve as the primary support system rather than the family. Identifying and communicating with the patient's *significant others*—the general term used by social scientists—can mobilize resources that help a hospitalized patient through acute phases of illness or gain their cooperation in helping a chronically ill patient accept and maintain preventive or therapeutic regimens.

CONNECTING WITH THE FAMILY

A recently married young woman decided to consult her long-standing gynecologist about family planning. Since she and her husband had several questions about how long they could delay starting a family without adversely affecting the potentiality for having children, the two of them appeared in the physician's office for the appointment. When he saw the husband, the doctor reacted very strongly; he refused to talk with them, saying he would deal only with his patient. The young woman argued with him, reasoning that since she was paying for the appointment, she should be able to use the time as she wished. The physician would not change his mind and the couple left. The young woman found a new gynecologist.

The reasons underlying this doctor's attitude were not made clear, but his actions do help illustrate a principle. Failure to take into account the role of a significant other, in this case the spouse, as a necessary participant in the primary patient's health care decision making was cause enough for the patient to terminate their professional relationship. While both the physician's behavior and its result may be considered extreme, the dynamics depicted are not at all uncommon; that is, ignoring or avoiding communication with the patient's family.

Identifying Who Is Significant

When a patient is admitted to the hospital, those who are most important to that person often can be found visiting. If patients perceive you as their primary physician, you frequently are introduced to parents, children, spouses, or perhaps others. At times, the family will approach you for information, reassurance, or even to complain. When dealing with outpatients, the physician is less likely to come in contact with an individual patient's familial network, unless you are treating several members of the family.

For all the reasons mentioned previously—assistance in diagnosing psychosomatic ailments, intervening in illness-producing family patterns, and mobilizing family resources—it is insufficient to leave data about significant others to happenstance. A fundamental portion of every initial history should contain such questions as the following:

- Are you living with anybody?
- If so, with whom?
- If not, who are the people you go to for help with problems (or, conversely, to celebrate good news)?
- What is a typical day like for you?

It may be important for you to explain that such information is necessary to arrive at a full picture of that person's state of health and health care needs. Asking questions like "How are things at home?" and "How are things at work?" should be a part of subsequent outpatient visits as a way of checking to see whether the individual's life situation and particularly the interpersonal support network has undergone any major changes.

Within reasonable limits, it is advisable that you be receptive to communications initiated by those who have been identified as significant, remembering that a single family member's illness has systemic as well as individual repercussions. Three exigencies typically prompt a patient's family members to interact with his or her physician: relieving anxiety, breaking bad news, and informing and decision making.

Relieving Anxiety

In instances ranging from concern over a spouse's blood pressure to panic over a child's laceration in the emergency room to care of a critically ill parent, the physician is often singled out, appropriately or not, as a likely source of assurance. The support-giving skills of empathy and listening that have been mentioned throughout this book are once again needed, though they may be put to use in a less extensive fashion. By hearing out the cause for concern, you may be able to correct a misunderstanding or refer the family to another member of the health care team who can more suitably deal with the problem at hand. A moment of kind attention from the physician, instead of an impatient or intimidating response, can be calming, even if there is little that can be done to change the focus of the family's anxiety. If you are unable to talk when the family approaches you, let them know that you are busy, but will be available to answer questions later at a time you specify.

Breaking Bad News

All practitioners eventually learn that anxiety cannot always be alleviated—the information you must convey can heighten tension and the patient's worst fear can come true. Communicating bad news can take many forms: announcement of death, birth defects, or anomalies; failure of surgery or medication to have the desired effect; or revealing permanent injury or progressive disease. Whether you knew the family members before the encounter, the task of bringing disappointing or unfortunate tidings is necessarily more than transmitting data; it carries with it the responsibility of also dealing with the human emotions engendered by your message.

It is best to be simple and direct in what you say. Using euphemisms or unnecessarily complicated terminology cannot take the pain out of the situation, but can unintentionally confuse or mislead. The Massachusetts General Hospital in Boston has addressed the issue of interpersonal techniques for obstetricians and pediatricians who deal with parents whose infants have been born with ambiguous genitalia. In this situation, the doctor must not only break shocking news, but must help the parents rapidly come to a decision about how the ambiguity should be resolved. As soon as possible after birth, the parents are made aware of the problem, accompanied by a simple explanation of how genital structures develop from indifferent embryo and how such development can be influenced toward more or less virilization. Once the parents have grasped the dilemma, they are referred within twenty-four hours to a center in which the staff discusses with them their degree of comfort with either gender role. It is made clear all along that physicians will supply as much information as possible, but final decisions are up to the parents. Initial surgery that shapes the outward appearance of the baby's genitals is performed within the next few months according to a schedule that depends in part on how difficult it is for the parents to live with the questionable condition. The presence of other siblings, grandparents, and babysitters may affect the decision. The communicative role of the physician in such cases is to give understanding and support to the family's inevitable confusion and dismay, then to facilitate a prompt resolution since it is considered psychologically unhealthy for the baby to undergo the onus of, and reactions of others to, ambiguity, and for the parents to respond vaguely to the natural inquiry, "Is it a boy or girl?" Such sensitive procedures stand in contrast to past practices of avoiding discussion of the problem with parents until the child reached age two or three (Crawford 1982).

You should be prepared to leave time for the family to react to whatever information you have announced. At least momentarily you are the most accessible object of response and may be the recipient of questions, grief, anger, blame, thanks, or even silence. Simple, human impulses are often the best on which to act. In the play *ER*, a touching scene transpires when a tough-skinned emergency room physician announces to a woman the sudden death of her husband. The physician-playwright, Ronald Berman, originally had the actor who portrayed the doctor explaining the technical procedures that had been used in vain to save the patient. The actor himself added the line, "I'm so sorry." A genuinely understanding attitude demonstrated by the doctor may not only comfort, but may serve as a basis for future interactions at less emotional times.

Informing and Decision-Making

The skills for information-giving have been discussed extensively in the previous chapter: use of appropriate, comprehensible language; sufficient explanation and detail; opportunities for the listener to ask questions; and referral to other sources, if necessary. The key issue becomes with whom and how much information is to be shared with the patient's family. At times, as with the previously cited case of the young woman and her husband who wanted to make a decision about delaying pregnancy, patients can be very clear about their desire to involve others in discussions of their medical problems. Others are equally as straight-forward in letting medical personnel know that they wish to keep knowledge of their problems to themselves. Such was the case of a forty-seven-year-old police officer who came in for treatment of a fractured elbow. Because surgery was indicated, a routine chest X ray was taken that, unfortunately, revealed a metastatic lesion in the lung. The man was adamant in letting his entire health care team know that he did not want any of the members of his family, specifically his wife and three adult-aged children, to know. In the next few weeks, the policeman's physical condition and appearance deteriorated, and several of his doctors were, indeed, contacted by the family. Because the patient's message was unambiguous in terms of the limits he wished to set on his family's involvement in his medical situation, his diagnosis and treatment were kept secret. (Three months later, his wife inadvertently saw his diagnosis written on a hospital admission form.)

The wisdom of this man's decision must be viewed within the context of his family relationships and his personal value system. Discussion of differences in judgment can be initiated by the physician with the patient. Should a female patient share with her husband the fact that she is terminating a pregnancy? An airing of both your own and her concerns on this matter can clarify the final decision. In other cases, the medical implications create impelling circumstances for you to try to influence the family network, as with a patient who hesitates in telling his or her spouse about contracting venereal infection.

Confidentiality of information pertaining to a patient is a sensitive and complex issue with legal and ethical ramifications that extend beyond the scope of this book. A general rule is to respect the confidentiality of the physician-patient relationship whenever possible by discussing with the patient what information can be divulged, to whom, for what purpose. As the medical advisor, you should reasonably attempt to influence such decisions when matters of health and recovery are at stake.

Involving Family Members

Much less frequently, family members and significant others are consciously considered by physicians as participants in a management plan. That such consideration is not more routine is unfortunate. Particularly for ambulatory patients with chronic conditions like heart disease, diabetes, and hypertension, the understanding and cooperation of those who live with or are close to the sick individual can be crucial to recovery, treatment, and prevention of recurrences of acute episodes. The family can be useful in reminding the patient to take or in helping to administer medications. Litman (1974) reports a special problem can be anticipated when the wife-mother in a family becomes ill. She traditionally has been the primary agent of health behavior in the family, the central agent for care and cure, and the family member most likely to take action in response to symptoms. Because of her pivotal role in the family unit, it becomes more difficult for her to be ill. Not only may she herself be reluctant to accept the sick role, but other family members may perceive her as less vulnerable and more indispensable to family functioning. Therefore, family members as well as the patient herself may need extra prompting from you to ensure that the patient receives proper treatment, rest, and relief from normal responsibilities when needed. However, a sign that sex roles within the family may be changing was noted by Gorton, Doerfler, Hulka, and Tyroler (1979). They found that fathers, while still maintaining ultimate authority within the family structure, are being more expressive and showing increased concern about daily activities in front of children and therefore may be more likely to play a role in molding children's illness behavior than has been assumed previously. This implies that you should more frequently consult with the husband-father.

In a more subtle sense, changes in life-style, work habits, and environment are difficult to sustain and are bound to affect the family as well as the patient. Because family members influence the perception and interpretation of symptoms, perpetuate the use of home remedies, try one another's medications, and encourage or discourage patterns of consultation with physicians (Mabry 1964), it is important for all involved to have a shared recognition of why change is necessary and what needs to be done. Such discussions also can dispel unfounded beliefs that may follow from a bout of serious illness in the family. Heart attack victims and their spouses, for example, may unnecessarily curtail sexual activities for lack of accurate information and mutual understanding.

Sometimes the entire family unit should be considered as "the patient." According to Baranowski, Nader, Dunn, and Vanderpool,

Certain health risks and types of health behavior—especially high blood pressure, overweight, smoking, use of alcohol, eating habits, and use of health services—are found to be highly correlated with family membership (1982, p. 162).

This research group found that a family-based intervention was particularly useful in providing emotional support for dietary change, though it did not work as well for modifying exercise habits. Gaining some background information about the way the family operates may be useful to you in terms of devising a family-based health care strategy. Child-rearing attitudes that recognize the child as an individual and foster the child's assumption of responsibility have been associated with such positive health behaviors as toothbrushing, proper sleeping habits, regular exercise, good nutrition, and refraining from smoking, while children raised in families with an autocratic style of childrearing are not as likely to practice such healthy behaviors (Pratt 1973).

THE PEDIATRIC TRIAD: PARENT, PEDIATRIC PATIENT, AND PHYSICIAN

Thus far, our emphasis has been on increasing and improving communication among physicians, adult patients, and the families of patients. However, when children are the focus of the clinical situation, doctors frequently address family members while almost excluding the young patient.

Medical students often refer jokingly to their pediatric rotations as "veterinary medicine," analogizing children to animals because of the perceived difficulty with communication. The usually integrated tasks of history taking and physical examination are frequently divided into a two-part exercise, the first with the parent and the second with child. Two assumptions that underlie this practice in pediatrics must be carefully examined. One assumption is that the parent or guardian is a responsible, astutely observant, and objective person who can intuitively translate the child's behavior into medically identifiable signs and symptoms. Although most parents are capable of doing a remarkable job in the care and understanding of their children, it is often expecting too much to think they can be so observant, intuitive, and objective in their assessments of their own sick children. A related issue is the common practice of taking for granted that the parent, usually the mother, who brings the child to the office or hospital is the best single informant, and then to rely on her exclusively not only during the initial interview, but in subsequent discussions of treatment. Even if one individual, such as the mother, is the best informant about the child, it may be critical to identify others highly involved in family decision-making, perhaps the father or grandmother, to discuss such problems as whether to do a spinal tap or perform surgery.

The second false assumption is that the pediatric patient is not responsible for, or capable of, giving information related to the problem or illness. This is an erroneous generalization that must always be considered in light of the individual differences among children. Understanding the developmental stages of communication is a useful basis for conversing with children to elicit information. For this reason, a brief review of the progression of verbal and nonverbal abilities is presented below.

Development of Communication Skills

The infant's acquisition of speech begins with throaty sounds at three to five weeks of age and progresses to "cooing" of vowel sounds at about three months. By six to seven months, most infants begin "babbling," sounds that consist of single and multiple syllables such as *baba, dada,* and *mama.* Over the next few months, infants will begin to produce sounds closely resembling ordinary speech, but devoid of conventionally ascribed meanings. This "jargon" phase, from the ninth to the thirteenth month, closely overlaps with the acquisition of commonly shared language. At this time, the astute caretaker will begin to associate a few particular sounds or "words" with tangible referents such as mother, father, brother, doll, or cookie. Although parental pride sometimes will facilitate the perception of connections between sounds and objects, it also should be understood that parents often have a wealth of experience with the individual child which enables them to understand many words that the outside observer would regard as mere babbling.

From one to two years, there is often an accelerated but highly variable growth in acquisition of new vocabulary. During this period, the toddler also begins to make characteristic gestures, such as waving the hand while uttering a sound to mean "bye-bye" or "night-night." It should be noted that the child's understanding of speech with the resultant ability to obey commands usually begins before he or she is able to speak. By the age of two, the average toddler can use 20 to 300 words, although studies have shown this range to vary from 5 to 1212 (Bawkin & Bawkin 1972). These words are primarily nouns used for people and common things in the child's environment. Verbs and pronouns usually develop more slowly after two years of age. The progression of language acquisition continues at a variable rate up to eighteen years at which point the average individual has a vocabulary of 14,000 words. However, by age four, children's syntax has matured to the point at which they can interact statisfactorily with adults (Wood 1981). Thus, *pediatric patients four years old and older should be considered as sources of information during the medical interview.* The amount of conversation that occurs in each child's home and school environment appears to be a major factor influencing communication proficiency, although general intelligence may have a gross effect on the range of linguistic ability.

Other behavioral observations and psychosocial theories can help us understand children. They often begin nondiscriminate smiling at three to six weeks, which progresses to smiling specifically at faces by three to six months. Starting at about seven months, children selectively smile only at those familiar faces in their surroundings. This latter period corresponds to the development of stranger anxiety from seven to nine months, when children first appear to be frightened by all but the closest family members. Stranger anxiety heralds separation anxiety from twelve to thirty months when children respond with distress and sadness when separated from their primary caretakers. Although separation anxiety is reduced markedly by three years of age, its effect continues to influence the behavior and affect of older children and even adults, particularly in such times of stress as illness or hospitalization.

A related developmental perspective is provided by Erikson (1964) in his description of psychosocial development. The infant first struggles with trust versus distrust, the conflict that is the basis for the development of stranger and separation anxiety. By the second year of life, this dynamic yields to the tension over autonomy versus shame when the infant tries to gain separateness from the parents by a contrary, constant use of "no" and by gradually developing skills such as walking, eating, and controlling urination and defecation. It is in this critical period that the toddler-to-be-adult acquires the attitude of "I'll do it myself," to which the physician must be particularly sensitive—the pediatric patient at this point is very aware of being ignored by the doctor. By the third and fourth years of life, the next developmental stage of initiative versus guilt appears, wherein preschool children continue to resolve the conflict over mastering their bodies and environments without feeling that they have overstepped parental authority.

Piaget (1974) has provided a final perspective in his observation of children's cognitive maturation. A few points are particularly relevant to observing and relating to pediatric patients. Infants make responses only to their sensory environments, resulting in reflexes such as grasp, startle, and suck. By age two, infants' thinking becomes concrete as they begin to associate sounds and people with things and events. "No" means to stop, the opening of a cookie jar means a treat, a bottle of milk triggers movement and noises that indicate they want to drink. Throughout the preschool and school years, children expand this concreteness into a desire to understand rules that benefit them in school and help them adapt to the norms and rules of their cultures. They learn to cross streets, play games, and manipulate numbers. As adolescence approaches, most young people acquire a sense of abstraction so they can understand more complex concepts that go beyond literal rules and regulations. Adolescents differ greatly among themselves in abstract capabilities. These differences will determine to what extent they will be able to understand disease processes explained to them by physicians.

Medical practitioners should also be aware of children's gradual understanding of death, which begins at age three or four and becomes more complete at age eight, which is perhaps best illustrated by the following story. Three brothers, ages four, six, and eight, were walking along a beach when they came across a dead seagull. The four year old remarked, "It's just sleeping. It will get up and fly away soon." The six year old said, "No, it's dead, but it might come back to life." The eight year old said, "No, it's dead for good. Let's dig a hole and bury it."

Interviewing Children

With the infant or toddler, it is advisable to address the parent first while watching the child's reactions. Because young children take time to warm up to the physician, this initial conversation with the adult will allow the child to feel more comfortable. When children see that their parents are not fearful or anxious in this situation, they begin to feel less threatened as well. This adjustment will help make subsequent questioning and physical examination of the patient easier.

When interviewing the parent or both parents, it is important to separate what they have actually observed from their subjective interpretations or speculations. This differentiation is essential and should be done tactfully to avoid creating the impression that you do not trust their reports or intuitive feelings. If a mother says her son had a fever, ask her how she knew this. You can then learn if she took the child's temperature with an oral or rectal thermometer, felt his forehead, or just assumed it because he was cranky or had a reddish flush to his cheeks. There is considerable variation in the way different parents use such terms as *diarrhea, croup,* or *congested* and their usage must be carefully assessed in context. When a mother volunteers a subjective judgment like "My daughter has an earache," it is important to note which behaviors led her to this conclusion; for example, the child was rubbing her ears, pointing to her ear and saying "hurt," or woke up crying like the last time she had an earache. When parental observations become more subjective or involve more assumptions, it is critical to take more care in evaluating the basis for the parent's interpretation. For instance, if a father repeats that his child has been restless and sleeping poorly at night, there are several possible explanations. A restless, tearful three year old suffering from nightmares, a stomach ache, or chills will disturb the sleep of most parents. Alternatively, an anxious, overly protective parent may be interfering unwittingly with the child's sleep by continually "checking."

When parents go beyond observation and assessment, physicians must be especially alert. Often parents do have an intuitive understanding of what is wrong with their children, but sometimes their own problems affect the situation. For example, a mother of a two-year-old boy presented to her pediatrician, complaining that her son was not eating well, despite the fact that the child's weight and height were normal and he appeared healthy. The mother then speculated that the boy was feeling badly since her husband's death three months before. Further questioning revealed that the mother herself had lost ten pounds in this time period and, in addition to losing her appetite, was sleeping poorly. The pediatrician's skill in interviewing allowed her to make a diagnosis of depression in the mother.

While focusing conversation on the accompanying parent may be a necessity if the patient is acutely ill, it is a dysfunctional strategy when there is a longitudinal relationship between physician and child. Although most physicians tend to include children over six in some portion of the clinical interview, it should be remembered, as previously stated, that younger children can make contributions too. A vignette of an actual case will illustrate this point. A mother and her three-year-old daughter came to the physician's office. The mother complained that the child was "acting strangely" and in a tearful manner expressed her fear that the girl was retarded. Upon further probing, it came to light that her niece had been diagnosed as having mental retardation a year before when she was the same age as her daughter. However, the mother became too distraught to give a more recent history. While the doctor attempted to let the woman calm down, he noticed that the child seemed bewildered and moved her head quickly at times, looking up at the ceiling. The physician asked the girl, "What do you see up there?" The child pointed up and said, "Birdie. Birdie fly up there." Observing the child's flushed face and interviewing the mother further revealed that her daughter had been given eye drops that morning by an ophthalmologist. The eye drops, containing an anticholinergic compound, had produced an atropine toxic psychosis in the child. Although it is possible that an astute clinician could have made the diagnosis without talking to the patient, her "report" of visual hallucinations was instrumental to a fast and accurate diagnosis.

With children between the ages of six and twelve, it is frequently useful to interview the parent and child together to obtain the fullest data base and then to direct further questions to the patient while performing the physical examination, making it a more personalized experience for the child. When the history and physical portion of the visit is complete, it is best to discuss your findings with both child and parent. Having children leave the room often arouses their concern and creates anxious scenarios in their minds. However, with very serious issues such as suspected diagnosis of leukemia or the need for surgical intervention, it is important to respect the parents' opinion of how, when, and who will discuss these issues with their child.

Whenever the physician suspects emotional or development problems, it is essential to interview both parents as well as other informants such as teachers. This issue must be broached carefully so as not to offend the parent who has brought the patient to your office. It is always important to be alert to both the verbal and nonverbal interactions between parents and children that occur in front of you. Such data help you evaluate psychosocial dynamics in the family, as well as possible obstacles to follow through on management plans at home.

> The more chronic the condition under consideration or the more it involves behavior problems, the greater the necessity . . . to communicate with the child alone for assessment and supportive help. (Carek, 1980, p. 2)

By speaking with the child alone, you also increase the opportunities for the patient to verbalize fearful fantasies about the illness or treatment, which you may be able to quell or at least deal with directly. Private discussions with the doctor may have special importance for adolescents, who are struggling with issues of incipient independence and sexuality. Unless they feel their conversations with you will be held in confidence, it is unlikely that they will cooperate in giving full histories or in bringing up the problems that are most pressing. One of the most difficult situations is the teenager who approaches the physician about birth control. It should be clarified with the patient whether the parent is aware of this request. While you should encourage children to be honest with their parents, the confidentiality of physician-patient communication should be respected. The physician's option to provide confidentiality when prescribing birth-control methods to a minor is now being hotly debated. Federal legislation may eventually dictate the physician's course of action in this situation.

Several research studies have focused on communication within the pediatric triad of parent, pediatric patient, and physician. The results, while variable, indicate definite trends that help us determine how to make such interactions more effective. Describing encounters in private pediatric practice, Arnston, Droge, and Fassl (1978) found the following:

- Physician and parents have a strong reciprocal relationship in terms of the types of communication used with one another. Specifically, the more affective or socioemotionally-oriented statements used by one, the more the other would respond in kind.
- While pediatricians tended to associate symptoms with environmental factors, parents tended to associate them with medication and professional treatment, instead. A separate study verifies this observation, noting that emphasis on environmental factors may make parents feel defensive, as if they are responsible for the problem at hand (Sharf 1979).
- The more experienced the parents are with handling pediatric problems, the less the doctors and parents talked about symptoms or were repetitious. While this finding seems commonsensical, there is an inherent danger that the experienced parent may assume too much and ask for too little explanation when circumstances are not routine.
- The pediatricians tended to be especially sensitive to the needs of parents who had endured past illnesses in the family.
- The more questions the doctors asked and the more symptoms the parents mentioned, the more the parents thought the physicians liked talking with them.

Observing mothers and pediatric residents in an emergency room setting, Korsch, Gozzi, and Francis (1968) and Francis, Korsch, and Morris (1969) noted that *cooperation* (these studies used the term compliance) correlated above all with the parent's degree of satisfaction with the communication that occurred with the physician. Satisfaction was more likely when a mother felt her expectations had been met, when her concerns had been elicited and respected (as expressed in the questions "What worried you most about your child's illness?" and "Why did that bother you?"), when she received feedback about her child's condition and progress, and when the physician talked with warmth and sympathy.

COMMUNICATING WITH GERIATRIC PATIENTS

Although children and elderly patients are markedly different, they have some similarities that require physicians to alter their typical approaches to establishing rapport and gathering historical and observational data. Both pediatric and geriatric patients are viewed as lacking such cognitive traits as memory, verbal skills, and abilities to think abstractly and to be adequate informants. Doctors thus feel they should interview relatives and significant others to obtain information. Second, both are perceived as not fully capable of carrying out detailed treatment plans without the help of others. Given that physicians approach them as if they were children, it is not surprising that geriatric patients often react negatively to these assumptions, feeling that their independence and autonomy have been slighted. Studies of elderly patients in treatment reveal that health professionals frequently violate geriatric expectations of quality health care (Hershman, Fritz, Russell & Wilcox 1981). These expectations include preferential, individualized care; empathic treatment; respect for the patient's opinions and self-assessment; and avoidance of derogatory labels. Perhaps more emphatically than in other clinical situations, effective communication with geriatric patients calls for awareness of their expectations of humane treatment, adaptation of messages to the individual within his or her personal context, and connections with the family network in such a way so as *not* to bypass the resources and contributions of the patient.

COMMUNICATING WITH PATIENT ADVOCATES

As was mentioned in Chapter 4, patients suffering from acute episodes of illness tend to be more emotionally needy and dependent, and less able to act on their own behalf than in more normal circumstances. A relatively new concept is that of a *patient advocate* to help individuals who are hospitalized and acutely ill. The patient advocate role may be filled by several different kinds of people—a hospital staff member specially designated to perform such duties, the patient's family physician, or a family member or close friend whom the patient has asked to act on his or her behalf. Although initially it may seem to be a nuisance for you to have to talk with an intermediary, the patient advocate may be able to discuss such emotionally laden issues as treatment choices or patient complaints in a calmer, more reasonable manner than the patient can presently muster. The presence of a patient advocate certainly does not, and should not, preclude direct communication between you and your patient. The patient advocate may well turn out to be a valuable asset to the physician-patient relationship by clearly representing the patient's point of view, influencing the patient's decision making or behavior toward cooperation, and helping negotiate differences of opinion between you and the patient.

COMMUNICATING WITH THOSE OUTSIDE THE "SIGNIFICANT" NETWORK

As nearly all medical practitioners have experienced, people outside the more intimate or significant circle of the patient may ask the doctor for information and reports on the patient's status. Requests commonly come from friends; extended family members; school representatives, including administrators, teachers, school nurses, guidance counselors and psychologists; and employers, presenting a host of legal and ethical dilemmas. Once again, whenever possible, you are urged to discuss questions of the release of information with the patient so that clear guidelines are mutually understood. When the patient does give permission to disclose data, it is important that you understand the purpose of the request so that you can judge the appropriate amount of detail to include. One sad incident that demonstrates this principle involved a ten-year-old boy who was referred by his pediatrician to a pediatric cardiologist. The two determined that he had a functional heart murmur, which of course has no serious consequences. The boy's school requested a physician's report. As a result of the report, which stated the medical diagnosis without elaboration, the school system took the precautionary measure of keeping the child from participating in any sports. This regulation continued throughout his high-school years. Following the completion of high school, he was drafted by the army. He reported for the army physical examination, thinking he automatically would be declared 4-F because of his long-term heart ailment. To his shock, he was found acceptable for the service, finding out at the same time that the functional heart murmur presented no threat to his health and that he had been unnecessarily prevented from taking part in sports throughout childhood. A slightly more informative report from the pediatrician to the school, as well as to the patient and his family, that explained the diagnosis in lay terminology may well have avoided this unfortunate chain of events in this individual's life.

Detailed verification by the attending physician proved helpful to a thirty-eight-year-old woman who had a positive reaction to a tuberculin test, but had negative sputums and showed no active evidence of the disease. Following the usual procedure, she was treated for the next year. Since she worked as a waitress in a restaurant, she was very concerned that her employer not find out her situation for fear of misinterpretation. However, word did spread around the community about her treatment and, as she had feared, she was told she would lose her job. Upon her request, her doctor issued a letter to her employer, explaining that her medical condition was not contagious and verifying that her state of health should not interfere or be hazardous to her work. The woman was permitted to stay on at the restaurant.

The physician's responsibilities in issuing information to outside sources is complicated, even when the patient makes an explicit request. There are situations in which it is preferable to exclude unnecessary detail, such as when employers ask for a letter about an employee who has missed work for a long time while being treated for mental illness, alcoholism, or other ailments that tend to carry social stigma. In such cases where discretion is of great importance, a brief note verifying that the patient has been under your supervision for medical treatment during the specified time should suffice. You also should forewarn patients that release of medical information in different forms to a variety of recipients could prove problematic. For example, a forty-five-year-old man, who had been hospitalized for depression and had been out of work for a month, asked his psychiatrist to respond to his employer's request with a purposefully brief letter that did not detail diagnosis or treatment. However, in the small firm in which the man worked, the employer also served as the insurance officer. Thus, when the physician filled out the insurance claim forms, which require a great deal of detail, the employer found out the nature of the man's illness anyway. In this situation it may have been preferable for the patient to have been direct with his employer from the beginning. Obviously, the situational factors surrounding a request for information need to be clarified with the patient before any disclosures are made.

SUMMARY

In Chapter 5, *network communication* refers to the patient's family and significant other friends and associates who might have reason to interact with the physician. Within the family unit, important events and the interactions among family members tend to influence any one individual's health care behaviors, states of illness, and treatment progress. Since family dynamics can be a crucial factor in the recovery or maintenance of a patient, physicians are urged to identify who is considered by the patient to be significant and to be reasonably available to these significant others for purposes of relieving anxiety, conveying bad news, informing, and decision making. Furthermore, situations are identified when the family should be actively involved by the doctor in treatment or prevention.

Due to the difficulty many practitioners have in communicating with pediatric patients, communication skills development in children is reviewed with implications for interviewing children and the parents. Hints for improving communication with geriatric patients are also mentioned. The notion of the patient advocate is introduced as a potentially helpful technique for physician-patient communication. Finally, the complications associated with information release, especially to nonsignificant others, are described.

As this chapter has begun to indicate, the more people involved in a communication encounter, the more complex and demanding of attention the situation becomes. In part, the complexity is enriching because each individual brings a different set of resources and creates new choices within the interaction. Concurrently, the opportunities for misunderstanding and unintended effects increase. With these thoughts in mind we will explore in Chapter 6 the modes of communication enacted among physicians and other professionals involved in medical delivery.

References

Arntson, P., Droge, D., & Fassl, H. E. Pediatrician-parent communication: final report, B. R. Ruben (Ed.) *Communication Yearbook 2*. New Jersey: Transaction Books, 1978.

Baranowski, T., Nader, P. R., Dunn, K., & Vanderpool, N. A. Family self-help: promoting changes in health behavior. *Journal of Communication*, 1982, *32*, 161–72.

Bawkin, H., & Bawkin, R. M. *Behavior disorders in children*. Philadelphia: W. B. Saunders, 1972.

Carek, D. J. Examination room conversation: a physician's perception. Paper presented at the Central States Speech Association convention, Chicago, April 1980.

Crawford, J. Personal communication, January 8, 1982.

Erikson, E. *Childhood and society* (2nd ed.). New York: Norton, 1964.

Francis, V., Korsch, B. M., & Morris, M. J. Gaps in doctor-patient communication II. *New England Journal of Medicine*, 1969, *280*, 535–40.

Gorton, T. A., Doerfler, D. D., Hulka, B. S., & Tyroler, H. A. Intrafamilial patterns of illness reports and physician visits in a community sample. *Journal of Health and Social Behavior*, 1979, *20*, 37–44.

Haggerty, R. J. Family crisis: role of the family in health and illness. In R. J. Haggerty and M. Green (Eds.) *Ambulatory Pediatrics*. Philadelphia: W. B. Saunders, 1968.

Hershman, P. S., Fritz, P. A., Russell, C. G. & Wilcox, E. M. Recognition of status norms among the non-compliant elderly: a communication course for nurses. Paper presented at Speech Communication Association convention, Anaheim, November 1981.

Korsch, B. M., Gozzi, E. K., & Francis, V. Gaps in doctor-patient communication I. *Pediatrics*, 1968, *42*, 855–71.

Litman, T. J. The family as a basic unit in health and medical care: a sociobehavioral overview. *Social Science and Medicine,* 1974, *8,* 495–519.

Mabry, J. H. Medicine and the family. *Journal of Marriage and the Family,* 1964, *26,* 160–64.

Piaget, J. [*The language and thought of the child*] (M. Gabain, trans.) New York: New American Library, 1974.

Pratt, L. Child rearing methods and children's health behavior. *Journal of Health and Social Behavior,* 1973, *14,* 61–69.

Sharf, B. F. A rhetorical approach to understanding the medical interview. Paper presented at the Speech Communication Association convention, San Antonio, November 1979.

Wood, B. S. *Children and communication: verbal and nonverbal language development* (2nd ed.). Englewood Cliffs, New Jersey: Prentice-Hall, 1981.

CHAPTER 6

Communicating with Other Health Care Professionals

In the seventeenth century, John Donne wrote that "no man is an island." Though Donne was making an observation about the human condition, his comment is particularly descriptive of modern medical practice. The hospital as a workplace requires physicians to interact with colleagues from a variety of specialties and with differing degrees of experience and training. In ambulatory, community settings, the range of personnel related to health care often expands, thus widening the circle of a doctor's co-workers. Private practice for physicians is moving increasingly toward a group model and even the solo practitioner needs to make ample use of referrals and consultations.

The need for increased communication among health care providers is impelled by several factors, which include a continual expansion in health-related knowledge and technology. The result is increased specialization, division of labor, and, consequently, a greater need for coordination. Simultaneously, the public is viewing the concept of health more broadly, thereby increasing the type of activities and practitioners that come under its rubric (Nagi 1975). This chapter will emphasize the skills needed for effective communication between colleagues. As you will see, these competencies are not usually taught during medical training and some even are contrary to customary physician behaviors.

COMMUNICATION WITHIN THE HEALTH CARE TEAM

A group performing surgery is often viewed as the model par excellence of a health care team. Everyone in the group focuses simultaneously on the same clinical problem or task, their goals are immediate and clear, each member's role is discretely defined within a mutually understood hierarchy, and a leader is unambiguously identified and followed. Even if interpersonal conflicts arise among team members, tensions usually are subordinated to the task at hand so that the quality of the surgery is not affected. Yet among groups of health care professionals that perform surgery, some work together better than others. In most other health care situations, circumstances are even more demanding upon individuals who are supposed to act together as a team.

The term *team* can have a deceptively positive connotation. Rae-Grant and Marcuse (1968) have perceptively pointed out many of the detrimental effects of clinical teams gone astray. For instance, an aura of "shared responsibility" can mean that no one is fully accepting responsibility or feeling accountable for the work of the team. Instead, there may develop a "covert conspiracy to carry on subtle forms of reciprocal alibiing and circular buck-passing" (pp. 4–5). Blurred roles and undifferentiated jobs may prevent each individual from working to full effectiveness. The other extreme is overspecialization, which can reduce interaction among team members and stop them from sharing pertinent information. The concept of team health care may become a mask that provides ways for members to avoid encounters with patients, a method of power and intimidation used to "bulldoze" patients into certain decisions, or an impersonal body that allows individual members to avoid facing their own feelings and inadequacies. Members may bring their own hidden agendas, such as aspirations toward personal prominence, that interfere with group goals. Even at best, it is time-consuming to maintain a team. While all these objections have some degree of validity, the costs and pitfalls of team health care must be weighed against the benefits.

Halstead (1976) reviewed all the medical literature from 1955 to 1975 in which a team approach to clinical problems was reported. Subject populations for the studies reviewed included patients treated for heart disease, hypertension, stroke, hip fracture, rheumatoid arthritis, diabetes, and comprehensive rehabilitation. He concluded that coordinated team care appears more effective than fragmented care for patients with long-term illness; the functional status of patients is improved or maintained, and there is improved control and less deterioration in disease activity when team care is given.

With this awareness of some of the advantages and problems inherent in the team approach to health care, let's now examine the communication variables that can make a difference.

GROUP GOALS

When a group of obstetrical and neonatal personnel assemble to perform an operation, they are well aware that their goal is the safe delivery of a baby. But once the baby is delivered, does this team have any responsibilities to facilitate the bonding process between parents and infants, or to teach patients proper self- and maternal-care methods? Obviously, there are no ready, preset answers to such questions. The answers will depend on the resources of the hospital, the philosophy of the obstetrics and pediatrics departments, and the knowledge and attitudes of the staff. In order for these activities to be operationalized in a consistent manner, they have to be acknowledged by all group members as objectives held in common. Therefore, it is important that team goals are clearly stated and communicated to all team members.

A second issue is who decides and defines what the goals are. In theory, one person—chief-of-staff, department head, or section chief—could set the objectives and inform the team, perhaps even in writing. Problems arise, however, when team members do not feel "ownership" of the objectives. Whether decisions are made by one designated leader, the entire group, or a smaller subgroup, effective team action will ultimately depend on the extent to which agreement and commitment exists among all individuals that comprise the health care team. Understanding and commitment require allowing those from whom cooperation is desired to question, exchange ideas, and suggest modifications. Furthermore, through discussion, conflicts between personal objectives and group goals may be identified and resolved before they interfere with clinical performance. One such common dilemma is the stated desire to eliminate unnecessary laboratory tests in order to reduce medical costs. While this may exist as a group goal for a health care team, physicians who are team members may individually feel that they are being pressured to omit certain procedures that would ensure the best possible diagnosis. Voicing such concerns, perhaps on a case-by-case basis, within the group may lead to mutually understanding what constitutes "unnecessary." Without active participation in formulating what and how tasks are performed by the team, it is unlikely that group members will adhere to the decisions that have been made.

A third issue that needs to be considered is how team goals relate to those of the larger organization. For example, while a health care team may strive to reduce hospital stays and avert further admissions for patients who can be taught self-care and preventive measures, the hospital administration may be attempting to keep its beds filled. Elucidating the goals of both the clinical and administrative groups can clarify points of conflict or demonstrate that working toward the clinical goals does not really interfere with actualizing those of the administration. When it is discovered that competition of aims does in fact exist within or among groups, then decisions to prioritize can be made.

MEMBERSHIP ROLES

In a general way, the terms physician, nurse, physical therapist, and social worker can be considered as roles, insofar as we expect people holding these titles to fulfill certain functions and responsibilities. Likewise, there may also be certain privileges, benefits, or liabilities associated with a role. Thus, expectations of what your job is exist for each of the other health care professionals with whom you work, based on their professional designations.

An individual may be perceived as filling another kind of role derived from an organizational context. For example, in addition to being a physician, a doctor may carry a label such as department head, section chief, attending, or resident. These organizational roles may qualify or add to the expectations that co-workers have attributed to the doctor role.

Finally, as a health care team carries out a variety of tasks together, it becomes evident that individual members are performing functional roles unique to the performance and maintenance of that group. Such group-related roles can be identified in any ongoing group, whether its task is medical care, laboratory research, or curriculum planning. Some members assume role behaviors that are pertinent to *task accomplishment,* such as the following:

initiating ideas	clarifying and elaborating
seeking information	orienting, giving direction
seeking opinions	summarizing
giving information	timekeeping, note taking
giving opinions	testing for consensus

Other members contribute by behaving in ways that *improve and maintain feelings of group cohesion and satisfaction.* Such process-centered roles may include the following:

encouraging contributions
compromising
keeping communication channels open
relieving tension
sharing feelings
observing and commenting on the group's own process

Occasionally, members will enact behaviors that are dysfunctional to both task accomplishment and group maintenance. You may recall individuals who engage in the following behaviors:

being absent, withdrawing
blocking or disagreeing excessively
seeking self-recognition
aggressing against or attacking others
dominating
joking excessively

These problems usually can be dealt with through group sanctions, including ignoring, confrontation, or encouragement. Discussion among team members can be useful in identifying the source of troublesome behavior. For instance, doctors often are accustomed to maintaining strong ties with their own professional groups (other pediatricians, other orthopedic surgeons, and so on). These connections may subconsciously or intentionally detract from that individual's relating well to an interdisciplinary group. Hearing other team members point out the repercussions on the group when a doctor avoids interacting with them may help the physician to better integrate.

Group functioning also can be hampered by overemphasizing either the task or maintenance dimension. In a group responsible for medical care, there is more likely to be excessive stress on getting the job done to the exclusion of attention to group process. Over time, this omission is likely to prove detrimental because the human needs and interests of group members are not being met.

One aspect of maintenance that presents an important issue for group communication is that of clarifying role expectations. How do you define your role within the team? What do you see as your responsibilities? However, answering these questions for yourself is not enough. The other team members must be made aware of your self-definition, as well. The next step is to check and compare how each of the other team members defines your role. Differences in perceptions need to be discussed until a mutual understanding of your role is established. The same process should be repeated for every individual in the group. It may be found that some expectations are simply not compatible or that one person cannot possibly meet all existing multiple expectations. Obviously, the business of clarifying roles takes extra time and effort; realistically, it is not an event that can occur repeatedly on a regular basis. On the other hand, clarifying roles is necessary when there have been changes in membership or tasks, or when disagreement over roles is causing problems in delivery of health care. For instance, it should be decided within the group who is responsible for communicating information to the patient. Consider the case of a twenty-nine-year-old male hospitalized for gastrointestinal distress. While the patient was being prepared for a gastroscopy, the laboratory reported to the nursing station that the patient's hematocrit level had dropped from 45 to 31 in the four hours since his admission. The supervisory nurse phoned the treating internist at another hospital. He ordered that a blood transfusion be started and said he would be there as soon as possible. The nurse began to carry out the order, but the patient became quite anxious, wanting details of his situation. The nurse herself was uncertain whether it was within her proper role to answer the patient's questions in the absence of the physician.

Conflict also may stem from a member's role expectations within and outside the medical care group. Medical students sometimes find during clerkship experiences that fulfilling their patient care responsibilities as a member of a health care team interferes with the responsibilities of the student role, such as attending lectures or using the library. In other cases, administrative, research, or familial obligations may adversely affect an individual's anticipated performance within the group. Once again, discussion among group members can be helpful in increasing understanding, lessening hostility, and perhaps shifting role responsibilities.

LEADERSHIP

You may be wondering why the term *leader* has not been mentioned as one of the very important, functional group roles. But what specific behaviors does a leader exhibit? The answer to this question is as varied as the possible range of personal styles and group needs. The one a health care team may call its leader may be a person with the most prestigious title, the greatest technical knowledge, the most personal experience, or the best ability to coordinate activities or deal with human relations.

Physicians are trained to take charge and give orders; in short, you are accustomed to being a leader. Furthermore, other types of health care professionals are accustomed to following the directives of doctors. Such traditional patterns are not always beneficial to the working of a team. Often blind obedience to a physician results in overemphasizing medical issues, lacking shared commitment to decisions, and less sharing of information (Rubin & Beckhard 1972). In a community setting, other personnel may be in a better position to give overall direction (Beckhard 1972).

Effective group leaders are usually able to mesh their own personal resources with the necessities of the task at hand and the dynamics of the group. Thus, a formal title may designate a person as leader (for example, chief, supervisor, or director) but unless the rest of the group accepts that individual, the issue of leadership is really unresolved. Bormann and Bormann (1972) explain that in the initial stages of a newly formed group, members "audition," showing what they can do for and within the group. Over time, various people are eliminated from leadership contention, until only a few, perhaps two or three, remain. Therein a struggle for leadership, overt or covert, ensues until the rest of the group throws its support to one or the other. For this reason, someone with the title of leader should not be surprised to encounter challenges from other strong members. If for some reason the leadership contest is not resolved and the formal leader does not gain the informal support of team members, people may still obey "the boss" because of a variety of motivations, but the performance of that team is likely to be hampered.

The terms *leader* and *leadership* are not necessarily synonymous. The former implies a particular person while the latter quality may be embodied in a variety of ways within a group. Although one person may hold or be acknowledged with a nominal title, the leadership functions— the essential task and maintenance behaviors necessary to effective medical care—are frequently dispersed throughout the membership. Or for the health care team with a variety of tasks to perform, leadership may shift among several individuals, depending on who has the most knowledge and skill for the job at hand. It is essential to realize that there can be no leadership without followership. Thus, part of contributing to team accomplishment is the capacity to follow the directions of another member who has acquired the group's support to take charge. By virtue of their socialization, physicians sometimes have difficulty being able to follow.

A CASE FOR CRITICAL CARE: PHYSICIAN-NURSE COMMUNICATION

Perhaps the most glaring incidence where neither leadership nor followship fulfill their potentials is the communication between physicians and nurses. Several historical differences between the two professions are responsible to a large extent for the difficulties that have evolved in their relationship. First is the basic sex difference that is only now changing. The predominance of male doctors and female nurses, coupled with traditional societal norms, have led to the doctor not only assuming leadership, but also maintaining an authoritarian posture that severely minimizes relationships and tends to limit communication to oral commands and written orders. Second, until the last decade, nurses have had markedly less general education and training, often in nondegree diploma schools. This factor also has played a key role in one-sided communication patterns.

Nurses, however, have come a long way. Many nurses now have advanced training as clinical nurse specialists, nurse practitioners, and have masters and doctorate degrees of nursing, resulting in changed interaction patterns in doctor-nurse relationships. Although many physicians lament these changes, claiming that "good bedside nursing" is no longer available to patients, in some situations these changes have resulted in a clarity of roles and communication functions. For example, nurse practitioners often have a clear written policy of what they can do in terms of history-taking and physical examination, as well as a specific set of dispositions they can make and which situations require physician consultation. These guidelines may lead to more limited, but satisfactory dialogue between nurse and physician.

On the other hand, not all changes have been for the better. Stein (1967) describes the "doctor-nurse game." The rules of this game dictate that nurses must find ways to make suggestions about patient care in a style that does not cause the physician in charge to lose face; that is, nurses cannot directly relate suggestions. Nurses face double jeopardy if they are not good game players. Those who do not contribute ideas are labeled as dumb and may sooner or later be dismissed; those whose ideas are stated too forthrightly or forcefully are begrudgingly considered valuable, but overbearing and difficult to work with. A few decades later, the rules of the game seem still to be in operation: doctors lead, nurses follow. In situations where nurses have developed expertise in intensive care settings to the extent that they are often more knowledge-able and experienced than house officers assigned to the unit, the nurses commonly discuss how to preserve the doctor's egos while simulta-neously maintaining their own dignity and concern for patient care. Whether a resolution or impasse develops in response to this conflict often depends largely on the relationship pattern between the chief nurse and the attending physician.

Because of the stress that physicians must face daily, it is easy to lose sight of the particular demands—some of which are created by physicians—that are put on nurses. Ley and Spellman (1967) showed that physicians spend 75 percent of their nonpatient "talk-time" on the ward talking with one another. The remaining 25 percent is spent almost exclusively with nurses. By contrast, nurses spend only about 40 percent of their nonpatient "talk-time" with each other, 30 percent with physi-cians, and the remaining 30 percent with other personnel. They are then in the unenviable position of having to communicate the physicians' thoughts and plans to a variety of people who often feel resentment toward the nurse, either because of what she says or the mere fact that she is telling them. Similarly, Grant (1980) found that nurses are the recipients of exceedingly high numbers of angry messages each day, 20 percent of which come from physicians. She demonstrates that aliena-tion which comes as a reaction to these angry messages is highly correlated with the annual large turnover rates of RN staff.

Good interpersonal practices employed by physicians can help counteract these negative interaction patterns, as well as upgrade the quality of patient care. You should periodically ask floor nurses what their views are on a given patient, sit with a group of them when they have their morning or evening report, and invite them along when you talk with a problem patient. For their part, nurses also must learn to exercise assertiveness in inquiring about treatment plans and in voicing opinions, even when they disagree with the physician. These personal behaviors ultimately can improve the current less-than-desirable state of physician-nurse communication.

DECISION MAKING

The Wholistic Health Center in Hinsdale, Illinois, an ambulatory facility located on the grounds of a church, puts a good deal of emphasis on prevention as well as treatment of disease. It is staffed by a family practitioner, nurses, a counselor, and a minister. Decisions about patient care are made with all team members in collaboration. The rationale for this arrangement is that health is comprised of physical, psychological, and spiritual aspects. This format of decision making fits both the philosophy and goals of this health care organization (Tubesing 1977). It would *not* be suitable for the type of health care administered in an emergency room.

Decision making can take many forms: consensus, majority rule, authority rule, even default or lack of response. Whatever the process, it must be appropriate to the task at hand (Rubin & Beckhard 1972). Decisions should be made by those with functional authority, those who have the best information and knowledge and are closest to the problem to be solved. The pattern that has been referred to throughout this chapter—physicians acting as solo decision makers in contrast to other health care workers who await doctor's orders—is often useful for the emergency and operating rooms. In many situations, the efficiency that comes with authority rule is gained at the expense of leaving the working group short of both information and commitment. In ambulatory settings, lack of participatory discussion leading to decisions and actions lays the foundation for the unwise separation of physiological and psychosocial pools of information. Such lack of collaboration could prove disastrous for community health centers attempting, for example, to aid families of patients with sickle-cell anemia or diabetes. Decision making for this kind of care requires identifying who will take responsibility and how best to handle the patient's emotional state, genetic counseling, early screening and diagnosis, treatment of acute episodes, long-term management, and patient education (Beckhard 1972).

NORMS

Every group that works together develops after awhile characteristic ways of relating and getting the job done. As a result norms or implicit rules set boundaries for members' behaviors. When norms are violated, groups typically act to reprove the offender in blatant or subtle ways. Norms can range from the degree of tolerance for late attendance to the way in which responsibilities are assigned and accountability is noted.

When a group finds itself bogged down for unknown reasons, it is often useful for team members to discuss the norms explicitly in order to identify those that may be interfering with the group's ability to do its work.

Rubin and Beckhard (1972) have repeatedly observed among health care teams norms that are dysfunctional to group performance:

- In making a decision, silence means consent.
- Doctors are more important than other health workers. Therefore, co-workers should not disagree with them; instead, they should wait for the physician to lead.
- Conflict is dangerous.
- Positive feelings, praise, and support are not to be verbalized. All professionals are here to get the job done.

Usefulness of Conflict

In order to understand why these sorts of norms are detrimental to health team functioning, let's briefly examine a model of healthy group development. Tuchman (1965) represents functional group evolution in four, easy-to-remember steps: *forming, storming, norming,* and *performing.* Forming describes the initial stage of a team when members first come together. It is a time marked by uncertainty because there is no mutual definition of the task and individuals wonder how they will be able to contribute and if they will be accepted by the others. Bormann and Bormann (1972) call this feeling "primary tension." The group moves into "secondary tension" or the storming phase when they begin to argue over goals, dimensions of the task, and division of labor. Storming indicates that team members are struggling to assume roles and achieve leadership. The norming phase occurs when these matters of contention are resolved and consistent group work patterns emerge. In a well-functioning group, members start to feel more cohesive and experience satisfaction in their interaction. More references to "we" in contrast to "I" can be heard. A group that continues to enact these sorts of trends is able to perform its job using the resources of all its members. Rewards are obtained both through well-coordinated task accomplishments and enjoyment of personal relationships among members.

This model is rich in implications for the analysis of group growth and problems. The point we wish to emphasize here in relation to the health team norms previously cited is that *conflict is a normal, in fact, necessary part of group development.* Teams that avoid or repress the storming stage are sometimes said to be "on a honeymoon". They are, in effect, stuck at an immature stage of growth that prevents a high quality of performance. Likewise, conflict that repeatedly occurs with no resolution of content issues, leadership struggles, or interpersonal antagonisms indicates another form of arrested development. For these reasons, silent members must be encouraged to participate; despite professional designations, health care co-workers must have the freedom to express disagreement in appropriate circumstances; and reactions to group process must be communicated at times, in addition to discussions focused on matters of task.

Language

Earlier in this book, it was pointed out that the technical language of medical practitioners often creates problems in the communication that takes place between physicians and patients. Damage also occurs when linguistic abuse becomes a norm among health care professionals. Christy (1979) has chided fellow physicians that "English is our second language," now replaced by what he has dubbed "Medspeak." Examples of Medspeak abound. According to Wish (1979, p. 507) symptoms become symptomology, swelling is edema, no change in medical condition becomes zero delta, and patients are bronked (undergo bronchoscopy), cathed (undergo catheterization), or scoped (undergo endoscopy). In addition to massacring the conventions of the English language, such specialized vocabulary and grammar fulfills the needs of individuals to appear learned, to be brief, and to hide what one does not know for sure (Christy 1979). What Medspeak does not do is to clarify meaning and facilitate understanding. In fact, a dialect of Medspeak that arises from practitioners of one particular subspecialty may prove unintelligible to health professionals who work in other subspecialties.

Curiously, however, if the inbred language is mutually understood within a specific group of individuals, it can function as a norm that in a sense enhances the group life of a health care team. This phenomenon is vividly illustrated in the verbal expressions of black humor that characterize the realistic novel, *The House of God* (Shem 1978). In the book's description of the medical internship in a prestigious academic hospital, language becomes the cutting edge between healthy cynicism and crude depersonalization of patient care. GOMERs, an acronym for Get Out of My Emergency Room, are pitiful, elderly patients, who are scarcely regarded as human beings, but who, in reality, are old folks with problems who continually frustrate the young doctors because they never get well and never die. We have heard such patients also called "bed plugs," in that their major activity is taking up space. According to the novel's antihero resident, the main thrust of modern medicine is to "turf" patients, especially GOMERs, that is, transfer a patient who has been admitted to your supervision to someone else's service. A step above GOMERs, according to the residents, are LOL IN NADs, Little Old Ladies in No Apparent Distress. These expressions are not simply the cruel creations of this novelist; they may be heard in teaching hospitals across the country. Although the use of such language seems to have the unfortunate consequence of increasing distance between physician and patient, it simultaneously does serve the very necessary and constructive function of creating cohesiveness and identity among the health care team.

That language is a key to group identity was recently made clear when an outpatient in a general medicine clinic amazed the health care professionals present during her narration of her history. She complained of having "a fever of unknown origin" and "pain in the right upper quadrant"; furthermore, she guessed (incorrectly, it turned out) that the seizures she was experiencing might be due to "tuberous sclerosis." This patient had violated the norms of patienthood by adopting the customary lingo of the clinicians!

Another aspect of language use that often can provide insight into the dynamics of a working team comes from what may seem a surprising source, namely, jokes, anecdotes, and dramatized stories. Bormann (1972) labels this material "fantasy themes" and theorizes that a story or joke is of particular significance when it "chains out," or catches on among group members, is referred to repeatedly, and becomes part of the group's history. The function of fantasies is to provide enjoyment of the group experience, give comic relief from tension, or deal indirectly and analogically with immediate group problems that are too sensitive or threatening to be confronted in a straightforward manner. Thus, quite serious feelings, such as anger, grief, or fear, may find outlets in a group's characteristic bantering, gossip, or humor. The surgical team portrayed in the television series "M*A*S*H" is especially adept in using language in this way.

COMMUNICATION FLOW

It should be clear by now that members of a health care team, those people involved in coordinated efforts to meet mutual goals of patient care, need opportunities to exchange information, opinions, and feelings. Whenever possible, face-to-face interaction is most effective because that format allows for feedback to occur, conflicts to be resolved, insufficient data base or misinformation to be revised. Just as environmental factors are important to good physician-patient communication, so a comfortable meeting room, as free as possible from distractions, will facilitate team communication. It is best if seating is arranged so that every member can see every other member's face and no individual is placed in a physical location that makes it difficult to be seen or heard.

In terms of information flow, it is necessary that all group members involved with patient care share a common base of understanding the problems and treatment plans. The more health professionals a patient is in contact with, the more important this rule of thumb becomes. A patient admitted to the hospital for a slipped disc could conceivably be seeing a family practitioner or internist, an orthopedic surgeon, a neurosurgeon, a physical therapist, and nurses concurrently. Having heard many horror stories about this condition, the patient is anxious to press any and all of the aforementioned professionals with questions about traction, surgery, length of stay in the hospital, and so on. Without a coordinated review of such a case, the patient is likely to receive a plethora of conflicting answers. Because it is not always possible to have face-to-face discussions with all health professionals involved in the care of one patient, the notes in the chart must be detailed, up-to-date, and clearly expressed. A sixteen-year-old girl was in the hospital for observation of endocrinopathy and treatment of depression. Because her physician had prescribed a monamine oxidase inhibitor, the patient had been carefully instructed about the foods, including yeast, from which she should refrain while receiving the medication. Unfortunately, the same message was not conveyed to the dietician. The patient thus became enraged when she received a tray with several pieces of bread and other off limits food items. The end result for communication flow in a health care team should be that pertinent information is available to all members.

*Charting as a Communication Medium**

In theory, the written chart for a patient should be a way of sharing information among numerous health care team members who may work different shifts or feel too pressured by time constraints to have meetings. In reality, the chart usually proves a less than satisfactory medium of communication.

---

*For much of the information discussed here on the patient chart, the author would like to acknowledge *Communication and the Chart,* a symposium presented at the University of Illinois at Chicago, Health Sciences Center, March 3, 1982.

One major problem with charting is attitudinal. It is regarded by many health professionals as cumbersome, a final task that is unrelated to patient care. For most personnel who use it, the chart is seen as a legal document, a record for self-protection. This certainly is a pragmatic and legitimate purpose, but one that elicits a different response than if communication was perceived as the main goal. Even as documentation, for legal purposes or research, the chart is often not kept up-to-date or is missing important pieces of information. Handwriting is frequently illegible, thus frustrating staff members who diligently attempt to read through the comments. A more pervasive issue is that health professionals, particularly physicians, tend to ignore the notes of others except perhaps notes written by those in their own discipline.

There are some steps that can be taken to make the patient chart a more effective means of communication. If the description in the chart is viewed as data for initial assessment rather than the final word, then the chart should serve as a stimulus for interprofessional interaction. Page and phone numbers should be included along with the signature to one's entries to facilitate follow-up inquiries from other members of the team. Second, the format of the chart notes can be altered to encourage more complete information, including the type of care administered, problems that have been encountered, and, most important, detailing of the thought processes of the staff person making the entry. It has been suggested that there be a central place in the chart for a combined major problem list to prevent fragmentation of medical psychosocial issues. Eventual computerization of the chart will eliminate handwriting problems, increase efficiency, and help routinize a fuller data bank.

No Substitute for Talk

Even when improvements in the charting system have been made, it is very clear that the written record—even a well-documented written record—is not a substitute for face-to-face communication among members of the heatlh care team. Because it is never certain who will read the chart, health professionals are reluctant to write down issues that may require confidentiality, such as rape, marital problems, or child abuse. The chart cannot ensure interprofessional collaboration regarding problems, treatment modes, short- and long-term goals and planning. Furthermore, it is difficult to convey feelings of subjective perspectives within the chart. There is a false sense of security in placing a critical piece of information, such as allergies to medication or food, in the chart and assuming the proper person will get the message.

Thus, we return to emphasizing the need for more regular team meetings. Though these take up valuable time, in the long run the amount of information shared may compensate for the time spent. Another method of increasing team interaction is for other health professionals, such as the nurse, pharmacist, and dietician to accompany physicians on regular morning rounds. Obviously, this alternative is less feasible in private settings where there are many physicians seeing patients throughout different hospital units. When such rounds do occur, physicians and allied health staff have an opportunity to talk, share opinions, and seek clarifications. Equally useful is the possibility of carrying on doctor-nurse-patient dialogues, doctor-physical therapist-patient dialogues, and so on, which can be an extremely positive force in minimizing confusion. Another commonly employed strategy is periodic "chart rounds" in which one or more physicians attend with the nursing staff and other health professionals. During these meetings, management plans for each patient are reviewed with various staff providing input.

Not to be disregarded is interpersonal conversation between individuals, either by phone or face-to-face. Since you will find that most allied health professionals are willing to talk with one another and, especially, with you, doctors need to exhibit more willingness to take part in these kinds of conversations.

Some frequently recurring questions relating to team interaction that need to be addressed include the following:

- Who decides what services, in addition to medical, are to be administered to a patient, by whom, when, and on what basis?
- Who will coordinate follow-up services after hospital discharge?
- Who is responsible for calling team meetings, either on a regular or ad hoc basis?

In a cohesive group that performs well, members need to be valued for the unique contributions each can make toward achieving team goals. To limit people according to stereotypic expectations of their occupational designations wastes team resources. As a functional team member, you have to be able to share the care of your patients; to learn from and teach others.

COMMUNICATION AMONG PHYSICIANS

So far, the discussion has centered on health professionals working in an interdisciplinary team format to provide medical care to patients. Frequently, physicians collaborate in other configurations which, though not in concert, still require thoughtful communication. When it comes to making referrals and arranging consultations, interaction between the physicians involved is sometimes sacrificed in the interest of time; the issue of communication may never even be consciously considered. Let's examine some familiar situations with unfamiliar attention to the interphysician relationships.

Detailing Requests

A very common scenario is the patient who is referred by one physician to another for an assessment of a problem. Primary care physicians frequently make such referrals to specialists. Referrals should be made through personal contact between the two physicians. It is imperative that certain basic issues be covered during the conversation.

> What specifically is it that the referring physician wishes from the colleague?

Let's say that an internist discovers one of his patients has an arrhythmia and decides to send the patient to a cardiologist for a consultation. What he needs to specify is that he wishes a recommendation for a treatment plan so that he can continue to manage the problem and care for the patient. This brings up a second important issue:

> Once the referral or consultation takes place, who is going to take charge of treatment?

It is important that all three parties understand the answer to this question. If it has not been made clear, the cardiologist may easily construe that supervision of the patient is now his job, while the first internist expects the patient to return for continued care. If the patient is confused, he or she will not know whom to call if the symptoms worsen or a crisis arises. Furthermore, patients should know *why* they are being referred. It could be a rude awakening for a patient who has complained of persistent stomach distress to discover the specialist his or her internist has referred him or her to is a psychiatrist!

Establishing Primary Authority

The question of who is actually in charge can sometimes become problematic, especially in the hospital. Not only are patients often confounded when they are seen by an attending physician, several residents, and a medical student; nurses may be put into very difficult situations if lines of authority have not been clearly drawn. In these circumstances, hospital policy is needed. If the second- or third-year resident is designated as primary physician, as is often the case in teaching hospitals, the supervising attending should cosign that resident's orders. If there is a conflict in judgment, this is a signal for the attending to talk with the resident—not to write a conflicting set of orders that will create confusion for the nursing staff. Sometimes a patient will be seen by physicians from two different services; for example, a woman with sudden, acute gastrointestinal pain and high fever is admitted to a general medicine service. Both medical and surgical personnel are utilized in the attempt to determine the cause. If two sets of orders, both medical and surgical, are written, the primary physician from the medical service should cosign the orders from surgery. This method ensures at least a minimal amount of communication and coordination between the two services.

When primary authority has not been specifically designated to a particular physician, it tends to be assumed, sometimes with unfortunate results. Take the case of a fifty-five-year-old woman admitted to the hospital by her internist when she suffered extreme tiredness and shortness of breath. She was seen by a consulting oncologist, who diagnosed her as having chronic lymphocytic leukemia. Not only did the oncologist tell her the diagnosis, but he forged ahead in discussing a plan for chemotherapy with her. The admitting physician heard the news the following day from the patient. This same sort of scenario can be retold with many variations: patients scheduled for surgery or dialysis by an unfamiliar specialist before the admitting physician has been told. Not only do such happenings undermine the relationship between the patient and the primary care physician, but they prevent that practitioner from exercising his or her detailed understanding of the patient's psychosocial state, of how best to relay the information, of whether members of the family should be present, and so forth. Both the admitting and consulting physicians have a responsibility to determine who will take primary authority in the case.

Clarifying Prior Information

In an age when many individuals see more than one physician on a regular basis and are being urged to seek second and third opinions for special problems, it is not uncommon for a patient to receive conflicting advice. The fact that these issues may not be major, let alone life threatening, does not detract from a patient's confusion or concern. A common situation that frequently receives varying answers is when one should resume normal exercise following surgery or a myocardial infarction. When new mothers ask when to begin feeding their infant solid foods, they may talk to one physician who advocates seven or eight months and then see another who recommends cereal supplements at three months. A baby previously diagnosed by the pediatrician as having bronchiolitis, after a particularly severe episode, is brought by the parents to an emergency room, where the doctor on duty informs them that the child has asthma. Both physicians, in fact, may be correct insofar as bouts of bronchiolitis often precede the ultimate development of asthma. However, if this data is not made clear to the parents they may be left feeling distrustful of both practitioners.

On relatively minor issues not involving medication or surgery, a physician often will respect another colleague's opinion unless he or she feels that the other doctor is acting fraudulently or practicing very poor medicine. Therefore, it is important to elicit from the patient what they have been told by other clinicians previously. In the case of the infant brought to the emergency room with upper respiratory distress, the physician could have asked, "Has your child been treated for these symptoms before?" If the answer is yes, the next inquiry should be, "What were you told the problem was at that time?" Even if you feel that you do wish to give contrasting advice, you should explain that what you are offering is a clinical judgment or *opinion* based on specific reasoning, as was the advice given by the first doctor. In this way patients can understand that they have a choice to make, rather than leaving the situation perplexed or disgruntled.

Coordinating Clinical Activity

It is sometimes said that part of the role of the primary care physician is to coordinate aspects of a patient's medical care. It should be noted that whenever a referral or consultation has been requested, the opportunity for confusion and unintended effects is always present. For this reason it is important that *someone*, the likely candidate being the referring physician, take responsibility for helping the patient understand the resulting activity.

Unless patients understand why they are being seen by another physician, they are likely to have anxiety over the unknown. In hospitals, where the timing of consultative visits often is not planned, the consequences can be frightening. For example, when a fifty-two-year-old man entered the hospital for an elective hernia repair and presurgical workup, he revealed evidence of probable old granulomatous disease in the chest X ray. Having seen the X ray, his surgeon happened to meet in the corridor a colleague in pulmonary medicine and asked him to check the patient. The pulmonary physician stopped to see the man that same morning, before the surgeon had the opportunity to advise the patient on the probable benign nature of the chest X-ray findings. Naturally, the patient was both startled and alarmed when the pulmonary physician appeared and said the patient was to be examined for possible tuberculosis. The surgeon could have avoided this complication by talking with his patient prior to the consultation.

Of course, the ambulatory setting may breed similar problems. When her ten-year-old son developed knee pain following a game of ice hockey, the mother took him to the pediatrician who voiced an opinion that the knee was not seriously injured. The pediatrician arranged for the mother to take the boy to the hospital for X rays as a safeguard. At the hospital, the mother asked to talk with the radiologist who confirmed that the knee was not fractured, but stated that the child might have a rare bone disease. This response made the mother feel very concerned so she took her son to see an orthopedic surgeon who, in turn, dismissed the radiologist's judgment as not important and said that the boy's knee was okay. Because she felt caught in a dilemma, the mother returned to the pediatrician who promised to call both the radiologist and the orthopedic surgeon. Only after the pediatrician coordinated the varying information did the mother feel assured that no further investigation or treatment was needed.

While effective coordination of clinical activity cannot prevent a patient from having to face unwelcome results, it can be a useful factor in communicating bad news and helping relieve some psychological distress. Such was the case for a thirty-year-old man who was admitted to the hospital by his family doctor after he had been experiencing sporadic, sudden loss of vision in the left eye. The family practitioner sought a consultation from an ophthalmologist, but also discovered ketones and sugar in the man's urine. He thus called in an endocrinologist as well. The family practitioner arranged that all three physicians be present when he told the patient the diagnosis of retinal artery occlusion and diabetes. Not only did the patient feel the psychological support of the medical team, but his questions regarding treatment and prognosis were answered promptly and fully.

INSTRUCTION AS COMMUNICATION

Role-Modeling

A special form of communication among physicians is the tradition of clinical education that involves interaction among attending physicians, residents, and medical students. Much of what is learned during clinical rotations and the early years of residency training stems from the student's observations of more experienced health care practitioners, as evidenced by the medical school aphorism "see one, do one, teach one." With so many community hospitals, health care facilities, and even private practices now affiliated with schools of medicine and academic medical centers, the chances of your interacting with undergraduate medical students or residents are greatly increased.

From this perspective, your everyday clinical activities—examining and talking with patients, interacting with colleagues and staff, contributing to case conferences and reviews—take on the extra function of role modeling. In styles that may range from formal demonstrations of a technique to informal or subconscious illustrations of on-the-job problem solving, you are communicating to clinicians-in-training not only distinct fragments of knowledge and skills, but in a more general sense what it means to be a physician.

Engaging

In a revealing study of a junior-level pediatric clerkship, Foley, Smilansky, and Yonke (1979) observed medical school faculty communicating to students during teaching rounds, working rounds, grand rounds, lectures, patient management conferences, and journal clubs. Content analysis showed a strong tendency for instructors to supply factual information in lieu of structuring discussions that encouraged analyses, problem solving, and application of clinical data. Only 17 percent of the total interactions were categorized as questions to students. Furthermore, these questions asked for facts to be applied to cases, requiring a minimal degree of engagement on the part of the students. Foley and Smilansky (1980) conclude that teacher-student communication should not only allow more time for questioning, but use questions that encourage divergent thinking and verbalization of the student's thought process. In short, good role models and clinical teachers go far beyond supplying facts and expecting "the right answer." They actively engage student participation, reasoning, problem solving, and exploration. By the same token, effective instructional communication necessitates active listening, as well as speaking.

Sharing Affect

There are a number of key junctures in the education of a prospective doctor that evoke strong emotional reactions: the first human dissection in gross anatomy lab, the initial encounter with a patient, the first time a patient dies, the grueling call schedule of the surgery rotation, and so forth. The function of a role model, of course, is to show a way in which to cope with these events. But moreover—as in previously discussed communication situations with patients, families, and health care team members—the sensitive instructor recognizes students' emotional needs by allowing time for students to share affect among themselves. If a teacher also is able to share his or her own feelings and experiences, so much the better; in this way, the students can perceive not only what you do, but how you come to select these particular choices. In so doing, the instructor models the communicative skills of empathy and self-reflectiveness.

Giving Feedback

All too often medical students and residents proceed through their clinical education, only to be surprised by the remarks of their preceptors on written evaluation forms weeks after the clerkship has ended. There are several reasons the message is not given while the student is involved in the activity. Patient-care responsibilities frequently leave little time for talk between students and practitioners. As the aforementioned study of the pediatric clerkship shows, faculty seem to regard their major communicative job as giving didactic information, not providing information on student performance. Noting someone is doing well may be thought a nonessential aspect of instruction while telling students they are deficient in knowledge or skills is an unpleasant task that many instructors understandably wish to avoid or delay.

However, putting off the comments, good or bad, until after the rotation has ended creates many problems. Obviously the feedback comes after students are able to make revisions, and may be too late for students even to remember accurately the behaviors that have prompted the instructor's remarks.

- The best feedback, then, is *timely.* It occurs as close as possible to the event to be discussed, providing the recipient is in a reasonable state of readiness to understand what is being said. Students who are temporarily upset, angry, or excited may need to calm down before hearing your comments.

If the purpose of the feedback is to help a student improve or capitalize on preexisting strengths, rather than to pronounce a final judgment, it must be worded in a way that does not engender a defensive reaction.

- Effective feedback is phrased in language that is *descriptive,* not evaluative. Students will benefit by learning what is missing from their work and how to present the data in a more organized way; it is not enlightening to be told one's workups are "lousy." Commentary should be as *specific* and *concrete* as possible.

- It is wise to *limit* how much is said at one time. Too many comments on diverse topics will diffuse their impact. Concentrate on what is most important.
- Do not assume silence or nodding means that students have understood what you have said. Encourage them to respond, question, and clarify your comments.
- Use conference sessions to give *positive* and *negative* feedback. Students need to be encouraged about what they are doing well, as well as corrected for what they do not do well.

FORMAL COMMUNICATION: PRESENTATIONS AND LECTURES

So far, this discussion of communication with health professionals has emphasized day-to-day interpersonal relations. Physicians also are frequently called upon to present information and opinions to larger audiences in more formal settings, such as meetings of professional associations, research forums, and didactic lectures. Having authoritative knowledge of one's subject is certainly a first requirement, one that a physician-speaker can usually fulfill. However, knowledge of the topic in itself is not sufficient assurance that a message can be delivered in a way that is both understandable and interesting to listeners. The remainder of this chapter will be devoted to ideas for improving your formal presentations.

Identifying Your Audience and Purpose

Whether you are communicating in spoken or written form, the issue of whom you are addressing is fundamental to all other planning. Certain key aspects of audience analysis should be considered each time you write a paper or give a talk. This is especially true for speeches or lectures that are delivered repeatedly to a number of different groups. Without the small touches that reflect the unique interests of the listeners who are present, your talk is likely to sound canned or stilted. In thinking ahead about your audience, ask yourself the following questions:

How large an audience can I expect to have?
What subgroupings are to be found in the entire group (sex, race, age, professional, or subspecialty affiliations)?
How knowledgeable is the audience about the topic?
How interested is the audience about the topic?

What time of the day will the talk take place; how alert will the
audience be?

How familiar is the audience with my credentials?

What motivates the audience members to attend this occasion?

Conjointly, you must clarify for yourself what your purpose is in talking
with this particular group of people. Do you wish only to increase
understanding? Or do you want to persuade them to support a particular
theory of disease, mode of therapy, approach to health care delivery, or
the like? Or do you wish to go beyond gaining attitudinal support by
asking these people to change behaviors or take action? Defining the
audience and your purpose should serve as a basis for all materials—
facts, anecdotes, opinions, arguments—that you decide to include in
your speech or paper.

Getting Attention

A typical problem with many speakers and writers is that they
assume their listeners or readers are inherently interested in what they
have to say. The degree of natural curiosity and attentiveness that an
audience brings to your material will vary with the situation. A group of
physicians attending a conference in order to collect continuing education credits may be less involved than people coming to a community
lecture purely out of interest in the topic. In either case, the speaker has
an obligation to try to identify the initial mood of the audience and
increase its involvement from that point.

For this reason, it is important to plan an introduction that will
stimulate attention, set a tone for what follows, and prepare your
listeners or readers for your main points. Unfortunately, it is all too
common to hear lectures that break into the topic in a mundane and
abrupt manner, that depend upon the audience bringing itself to the
speaker's level of interest, rather than the speaker seeking to reach the
audience. Effective introductory statements are vivid, amply detailed,
perhaps even humorous. They are carefully planned to actively involve
the listeners or readers and set them thinking in a manner conducive to
what will follow.

It is the speaker's or writer's responsibility to make clear to the
audience why this topic is pertinent and important to them, or how they
are or will be affected by the problem at hand. Your initial remarks tend
to be remembered far better than much of the subsequent material. If you
fail to hold attention at this point, particularly if you yourself seem
unenthused, it will be very difficult to regain audience interest later.

Organizing Ideas

In presenting major ideas, we usually organize our thinking in one of two ways. Most of the time, people choose a *deductive* approach, beginning by announcing a general statement or argument followed by more specific explanation or supporting evidence: "Today, I am going to discuss the recognition and management of cardiac arrhythmias." This is an appropriate and efficient approach when your listeners or readers are well informed at the start, realize they have a stake in the subject, and are eager to hear what you have to say. Recently, Dr. Jack Geiger (1982), a recognized expert with impressive credentials illuminated by the moderator, addressed a medical center audience on the topic of "Medical Consequences of Nuclear War." The audience was self-selected insofar as students, faculty, staff, and practitioners had voluntarily taken an hour from busy schedules in order to attend. Thus, it was probably safe to assume that his listeners were inherently interested in, or at least curious about, his announced topic. Quite correctly, he proceeded in a deductive manner: Were a nuclear attack to occur here today, the effects would be so debilitating that little difference would exist between the dead and the "survivors." That idea being his major thesis, he continued to describe the three main sources of mortality and morbidity: blast, heat, and radiation. With the aid of vivid supporting materials, Dr. Geiger had no difficulty in capturing and maintaining the audience's attention, as well as demonstrating a progression of thought and line of reasoning that listeners easily followed.

Deductive reasoning becomes an ineffective method of organization when your audience has little previous knowledge of, no recognition of its own relation to, or undefined, ambiguous, or negative feelings concerning the topic at hand. In these situations the speaker or writer must work harder to get the audience absorbed and must find a way of reasoning together with that group of people. If ideas are presented *inductively,* starting with concrete examples, case studies, or analogies that progressively lead up to a conclusion in the form of a general principle, the effect is to deflect resistance and encourage involvement on the part of listeners and readers. If they can be induced to follow the logic of your specific illustrations, the chances that they will attend to, understand, and perhaps agree with, your overall thesis will be much enhanced. Let's look at how this form of inductive organization was put to good use. The admissions committee members of a state medical school were having a difficult time putting into practice a mandate from the state legislature to increase the number of disadvantaged Hispanic student admissions because they could not define what constitutes being Hispanic. They knew, however, that arguing with the wording of the mandate would bring opposition not only from the state representatives, but from local community groups. In presenting their problem in public, therefore, the chairperson began with a litany of individual cases that had come before the committee. A white American woman of Irish extraction claimed Hispanic ethnic status on the basis of gaining a Hispanic surname by marriage two months before applying; a man born in Taiwan, raised in Argentina, and living in Miami claimed Hispanic status by virtue of acculturation; an applicant born and bred in the Philippine Islands chose the Hispanic, rather than Asian-Pacific Island-er, designation because her grandparents had come from Spain. Follow-ing a series of these and other complex cases, the chairperson concluded with the argument that the legislative mandate was in need of revision and clarification. Both the lawmakers and community advisory groups set to work to change the wording of the directive to the medical school.

In essence, the arrangement of ideas and the reasoning that underlies the presentation of ideas are essential factors in whether the thoughts will be understood and accepted. Inductive organization is an underused format that often can prove more interesting and a better way of getting results.

Once the major strategy of whether to proceed deductively or inductively has been made, the *arrangement of subpoints* is an issue. A relatively fixed number of organizing principles exist by which we tend to order ideas. Although these are sometimes used instinctively, they are at other times ignored, resulting in presentations that seem haphazardly constructed and are difficult to understand and remember. Concepts may be organized chronologically, as in explanations of laboratory or clinical procedures; spatially, as often used in anatomy lectures; categor-ically or topically, such as the list of nuclear explosion effects mentioned above; or relationally, in the form of problem-solution, cause-effect, comparisons, or contrasts (Phillips & Zolten 1976). As you plan the ideas, facts, and examples that you wish to include in a presentation, you should simultaneously be thinking of how and why the parts fit together.

Once the organization of subpoints is clear to you, you must ensure that it will make sense to your audience. For this purpose, the use of *transition statements* is invaluable, especially for oral presentations in which the listener cannot review what has come before. A distinct transition lets the reader or listener know that you have completed one set of thoughts and are about to embark on another: "Now that we have an overview of the history of narcotics usage in the United States, we will examine in detail current legal constraints in the prescription of narcotic substances." Similarly, periodic *summary* statements reiterate the points you would like your audience to understand and remember: "Thus, the five drug groups used most commonly in psychiatric practice are anti-psychotic, anti-depressant, anti-anxiety, lithium, and sedative-hypnotics."

Developing Ideas

Once you have planned ways to capture attention and organize
your ideas, the next concern should be how to develop and support your
main ideas with detail. A common mistake for less experienced speakers
and writers is to skimp on explanations, descriptions, and evidence,
assuming that what is obvious to them will be equally so to listeners or
readers. In most cases, what others understand of your communication
will not be based on intuition or mutual expectations; but will depend
upon your use of clear, adequate supporting materials.

It is necessary to provide *definitions* of key concepts in terms that
are meaningful to your audience. The concept of megaton was essential
to Dr. Geiger's talk on nuclear war. He could have given a technical
definition that would have been precise, but not understood by most
listeners. Instead he defined megaton in terms of its geographic and
medical consequences. Then he reviewed the same sort of consequences
expanded, given the probability of a twenty-megaton bomb drop.

Examples are representative cases used to illustrate a general idea,
principle, or argument. The best examples are vivid enough to help
listeners or readers form a mental image. The more the speaker or writer
is able to personalize the examples to the audience at hand, the more
powerful the effect. For Dr. Geiger's audience at the University of
Illinois, the city of Chicago was used as a specific geographic illustration of a target for nuclear attack. Looking at an enlarged map of the
metropolitan area, his listeners were able to identify where they lived
and worked, and then heard to what degree these places would be
affected by nuclear consequences. The speaker described how familiar
city landmarks would be blown apart, how commonplace building
materials, furnishings, and clothing would be set afire by spontaneous
combustion. Although a colorful example is an excellent device for
actively drawing in an audience, you should be cautioned about its
vulnerability. When presenting an arguable proposition, one good
example can be countered by an equally good one in support of an
opposing idea. Therefore, other types of evidence or support may be
needed in addition to examples in order to make a convincing point.

A common form of idea development in scientific circles is the use
of *statistics*, numerical summaries of quantities of similar cases. From
these, relationships and probabilities may be interpreted. They can have
a force that one or a few examples do not, in that they significantly
represent a larger population. Because physicians tend to be readers of
scientific literature, even if they are not researchers themselves, they are
used to digesting statistical data much more than a lay audience.
However, even with doctors, there is a point of diminishing returns. This
is especially true of oral presentations in which the information is heard
only once, and cannot be reviewed and clarified. An overdose of
statistics can detract from the liveliness of a speech (or article) and

deaden the audience's interest. Thus, in oral presentations statistics should be chosen with care so that only the most essential and meaningful are communicated. Often it is useful to ensure understanding by showing visual aids that will reinforce the spoken information. Comparisons can sometimes be employed in order to make one statistic more meaningful to a particular group of listeners or readers. To state the amount of dollars allocated to nuclear defense technology may signify little—we have become accustomed to hearing about government budgets amounting to millions, even billions. However, if the communicator is able to compare that amount with the money designated for medical education, cancer research, and so forth, the defense allocation becomes increasingly meaningful.

One final type of supporting material to consider is *authoritative testimony*. Naturally, it is advantageous to quote from sources that your listeners or readers already recognize as credible and knowledgeable. When that is not possible, you should let the audience know what the source's credentials as an authority are. (Remember that Dr. Spock was often quoted by the antiwar forces during the Vietnam Era, despite the fact that his credentials as an authority were in pediatrics!) Like examples, authoritative testimony may be easily discounted or confused when contrasting testimony is brought to light. If your listeners or readers are sophisticated enough to know of opinions that differ from that which you are presenting, it will be to your detriment to ignore the opposition. Instead, you should anticipate the audience's thinking by dealing with the disagreement head on, refuting the opposing evidence as strongly as possible.

Delivering the Message

The last major element of an effective presentation is your own personal *style;* an aspect of both writing and speaking. Most of your communicative style is already developed. Your tendency toward formality, inclination toward humor, or ability to articulate well under stress are all characteristic of style. It is often unwise to depart radically from what seems natural for you, for example, to insert jokes in a talk when you rarely have done so before; the results seem artificial and stilted. However, you can add a degree of flexibility to your own style by considering what sort of relationship you would like to establish with the particular group of listeners or readers you hope to address. Do you wish to disclose personal information or maintain distance, proceed uninterrupted or entertain questions, narrate in the first or third person? These are examples of stylistic choices that are open to conscious deliberation and amendment. What primarily determines your style is your selection of language.

Oral presentations have the added dimension of your personal demeanor. We have discussed many nonverbal aspects of communication in previous chapters dealing with physician-patient interaction. Public speaking and lecturing can be treated as enlarged conversation. Most of the same principles apply, though they may need to be carried out in a larger or modified fashion. As in a one-to-one encounter, *eye contact* is very important in establishing and maintaining rapport. With a large audience it may be impossible to meet the gaze of every individual. However, you should be able to scan the room and make visual contact with individuals in various places. Although seeing an occasional yawn, frown, or open newspaper may be somewhat disconcerting, these are cues that let you know that something else—more explanation, a clarifying example, a transition to the next topic—is needed. Be cautious about writing out the entire text of a speech, lecture, or conference presentation since this habit encourages you to look down constantly at your notes. If you are familiar with the material you are presenting, a topical outline with statistics or quotations written out is a sufficient guide for a talk, while not tempting you to pay attention only to the written page in front of you.

Your *facial expressions* and *gestures* can enhance or detract from the content of your talk. If they call attention to themselves, they prevent your listeners from giving their full attention to what you are saying. More frequently, however, speakers fail to use their faces and bodies often or forcefully enough to enlighten their talk. Rigid stance, motionless arms, hands gripping the lectern, and deadpan facial expressions are all ways of reducing self-expression and the audience's interest in what you have to say. Lack of variety is often true of *vocal quality* as well. Remember that your voice is a resource that communicates connotative meaning through pace, volume, and tone.

Another consideration for effective oral delivery is how best to use *visual aids*. One rule of thumb is to make sure that the visuals do aid, not dominate, the presentation. It is not uncommon to observe scientific papers in which the listeners sit in a darkened room and watch a monotonous series of slides, charts, or tables accompanied by a droning, disconnected voice. This format becomes so monotonous that it can make some of the audience fall asleep and nearly obliterates any of the aforementioned personal qualities the speaker can bring to the presentation. Visual aids should be selected judiciously with the intent of supporting the spoken message. Particularly when showing tables and graphs, remember that a listening audience can assimilate much less at one time than a reader who is able to go back and review information as many times as is necessary for comprehension.

When showing visuals with a slide projector, overhead projector, or printed chart, make sure that printing and diagrams are large enough to be read by all audience members. Keep writing to a minimum, using short phrases or key words whenever possible. Visual aids should be coordinated with the spoken material to provide emphasis or clarification. There is often a problem in distributing a handout, putting up a chart, or writing on the board before the talk begins, because the visual material catches the attention of listeners before they know what point you will be making and may decrease their concentration on other parts of the talk. Finally, as you refer to visual materials on the board or a chart, remember to step to the side, point with the hand that is closest to your display, and remain talking with your audience, not to the visual aid.

Concluding

As in a patient interview, the last few minutes of a formal presentation are some of the most lasting impressions that the listener or reader will remember. The purposes of a conclusion are to summarize, reiterate essential points, and leave the audience in an appropriate frame of mind. In the case of Dr. Geiger's talk to which we have been referring, he concluded by asking audience members to take definite action by signing a prepared petition addressed to members of Congress to halt nuclear armament. This was a conclusion designed not only to underscore the main message, but to gain active commitment from his listeners. An abrupt or weak ending can undermine the previous efforts you have made, while a well-planned, emphatic conclusion can leave your audience with feelings roused, interest peaked, and active thoughts.

SUMMARY

Chapter 6 explores communication patterns among physicians and their co-workers. The concept of the interdisciplinary health care team is examined in terms of its difficulties and benefits to quality health care. Aspects of team interaction that are discussed include: the formation and sharing of group goals; perception of membership roles, with an emphasis on those that contribute to task accomplishment and group maintenance; leadership development, with a special focus on the leader-follower relationship between physicians and nurses; decision making; group norms, particularly the functions of conflict and language; and communication flow, with a comparison of the written chart versus face-to-face exchange.

Communicative skills important to the processes of interphysician referral and consultation include detailing requests, establishing primary authority, clarifying prior information, and coordinating clinical activity. Effective clinical instruction is also viewed as communication among physicians and students with emphasis on the importance of role-modeling, actively engaging students, sharing affect, and giving feed-back. Finally, the art of formal presentations, whether for lectures or professional meetings, is detailed. Identifying audience and purpose, gaining attention, organizing ideas, developing ideas, delivering the message, and concluding the talk are all basic elements in effective presentations.

This chapter has spanned a wide range of situations, calling forth communication skills needed for team health care, referrals and con-sultations, clinical instruction, and public presentations. The common thread is your relationship with colleagues and co-workers. The fabric you weave envelops your practice, reputation, and the welfare of your patients. It cannot be taken for granted.

References

Beckhard, R. Organization issues in the team delivery of comprehensive health care. *Milbank Memorial Fund Quarterly*, 1972, *50*, 287–316.

Bormann, E. G. Fantasy and rhetorical vision: The rhetorical criticism of social reality. *Quarterly Journal of Speech*, 1972, *58*, 396–407.

Bormann, E. G., & Bormann, N. C. *Effective small group communication.* Minneapolis: Burgess, 1972.

Christy, N. P. English is our second language. *New England Journal of Medicine*, 1979, *300*, 979–81.

Foley, R. P., Smilansky, J., & Yonke, A. Teacher-student interaction in a medical clerkship. *Journal of Medical Education*, 1979, *54*, 622–26.

Foley, R. P., & Smilansky, J. *Teaching techniques: A handbook for health professionals.* New York: McGraw-Hill, 1980.

Geiger, J. Medical consequences of nuclear war. Address given at the University of Illinois at Chicago, Health Sciences Center, February 2, 1982.

Grant, B. W. *Anger and alienation: Occupational communication hazards for nurses and other health care workers.* Paper presented at the International Communication Association convention, Acapulco, May 1980.

Halstead, L. S. Team care in chronic illness: a critical review of the literature of the past twenty-five years. *Archives of Physical Medicine and Rehabilitation*, 1976, *57*, 507–11.

Ley, P., & Spellman, M. S. *Communicating with the patient.* London: Staples, 1967.

Nagi, S. Z. Teamwork in health care in the U.S.: A sociological perspective. *Milbank Memorial Fund Quarterly Health and Society*, 1975, *53*, 75–91.

Phillips, G. M., & Zolten, J. J. *Structuring speech: A how-to-do-it book about public speaking.* Indianapolis: Bobbs-Merrill, 1976.

Rae-Grant, Q. A. F., & Marcuse, D. J. The hazards of teamwork. *The American Journal of Orthopsychiatry,* 1968, *38,* 4–8.

Rubin, I. M., & Beckhard, R. Factors influencing the effectiveness of health teams. *Milbank Memorial Fund Quarterly.* 1972, *50,* 287–316.

Shem, Samuel. *The house of God.* New York: Dell, 1978.

Stein, L. I. The doctor-nurse game. *Archives of General Psychiatry,* 1967, *16,* 669–703.

Tubesing, N. L. *Whole person health care: philosophical assumptions.* Hinsdale, Ill.: Society for Wholistic Medicine, 1977.

Tuchman, B. W. Development sequence in small groups. *Psychological Bulletin,* 1965, *63,* 384–99.

Wish, J. B. Correspondence to the editor. *New England Journal of Medicine,* 1979, *301,* 507.

Afterword

Like almost every other circumstance of contemporary life, the education and practice of physicians is in the midst of being revolutionized by computers. Computers are presently invaluable aids to patient record keeping and certain types of diagnosis and monitoring. Doctors can shortly look forward to a time it will no longer be necessary to memorize long, everchanging lists of pharmaceuticals or remember complicated drug interactions. Not far behind may be software that can formulate diagnoses or generate management plans on the basis of inputting problem lists. In fact, such software may also be available to the lay public who then can practice aspects of primary care with the help of their own home terminals.

However, there will always be certain dimensions of medicine that cannot be relegated to the computer. Preeminent among these is the therapeutic nature of the physician-patient relationship. The interpersonal qualities that you bring to your encounters with patients is an element of health care that can never be programmed onto a floppy disk or simulated on the patient's home terminal. It is for this reason that continuous awareness, assessment, and improvement of your communication skills should be an indispensable part of your continuing medical education.

INDEX

Aaku, T., 12, 26
Activity-passivity physician-patient
relationship, 28
Acutely ill patient, 40, 49; dignity of, 53.
See also Hospitalized patient
Adherence as communication goal, 5, 6;
discussion and, 7
Adolescent, 50, 63; communication with, 74;
maturation of, 72
Adult-adult relationship, 28; with ambulatory
patient, 39
Advisory-compliant physician-patient
relationship, 50
Affect sharing, 100–101
Aine, E., 12, 26
Alternate health care, 13
Ambulatory patient, 27–46; adult-adult relationship with, 28; communication with, 31–32;
coordination of treatment for, 99; examining
room environment for, 30; follow-up for,
39–40; history-taking for, 30; interviewing of,
33–34; maintaining rapport with, 36–37;
minimizing anxiety of, 32–33; motivating of,
39; mutual participation in care of, 28; office
environment for, 29; sexual history taking
for, 40–43; significant others and, 63
Analogy, 40
Anatomy of an Illness, 13
Anxiety, 12; coping with, 23; in families, 65;
minimizing, 36; of severely ill patient, 59;
sexual history taking and, 43
Arnston, P., 74, 79
Attention gaining, 103
Attitude: toward charting, 94; toward children,
69; of family, 68–69; influences on, 14; toward
nurses, 88; of patient, 12; of physician, 14
Audience, analysis of, 102–103
Audiotaping interviews, 43
Authoritative testimony in oral presentations,
107
Authority hierarchy, 97
Autonomy vs. shame, 71

Bad news, communication of, 58–60, 65–66
Baranowski, T., 40, 42, 46, 68, 79
Barnett, K., 20, 26
Barsky, A. S., 34, 47
Bause, G., 34, 47
Beckhard, R., 86, 89, 90, 110
Bedside manner, for hospitalized patient, 51–55
Behavior: of children, 71; empathic, 24, 26, 65;
and illness roles, 68; of medical team, 84–86;
modification of, 40; nonverbal, 18–23, 36; of
physician, 36; for sexual history taking, 41;
supportive, 23–26
Blane, H. T., 21, 26
Body movement as nonverbal communication,
21–22
Borman, L. D., 58, 61
Bormann, E. G., 92, 110
Bormann, E. G., and N. C., 86, 90, 110
Bowken, H., and R. M., 70, 79
Brozmann, R. A., 42, 47
Butt, H. R. A., 38, 46

Care vs. cure, 23
Carek, D. J., 74, 79
Cassata, D. M., 43, 47
Cassileth, B. R., 57, 61
Chafetz, M. E., 21, 26
Charting, 93–94; drawbacks to, 94; vs. personal
communication, 94–95
Chart rounds, 95
Children, 31; attitude toward, 69; behavioral
development of, 71; as information-givers, 70;
interviewing of, 72–75; language development
of, 70–75; as patients, 69–70; significant
others and, 63
Christy, N. P., 91, 110
Chronically ill patient, 29, 40. See also
Ambulatory patient.
Clements, P. W., 43, 47
Clinical health team, 82. See also Medical team
Closed questioning, 34
Closure in medical interview, 37–38, 45
Cogan, M., 10
Communication, 1–10; with ambulatory patient,
39–40; of bad news, 65–66; breakdown of, 2;
with children, 72–78; clarity of messages, 6–7;
with dying patient, 58–60; elements of, 2; with
family, 64; feedback in, 16; flow of, 92–95; of
genital ambiguity, 66; with geriatric patient,
75–76; goals, 4t, 5–6; in health team, 81–110;
with hospitalized patient, 48–60; importance
of, 2; improvement of, 2–4; instructions as,
99–102; interactional, 16–17, 17t; language of,
15–17; lectures as, 102–109; listening and, 8;
nonverbal, 18–23; with outpatient, 27–46;
with patient, 11–25; with patient advocate, 76;
in physician-nurse relationship, 87–89;
among physicians, 95–99; presentations as,
102–109; referrals as, 96; with severely ill
patient, 58–60; situational analysis as, 6–7;
traditional model of, 13, 16
Compliance, of patient, 14
Computers, 112
Confidentiality, 67
Conflict: benefits of, 90–91; of medical
opinion, 97–98
Connotation, 7
Connotative meaning, 16
Consent, 57
Consultations, 98
Cooperation: as communication goal, 5, 6;
coordination of clinical activity, 98–99;
discussion and, 9; vs. compliance, 14
Cousins, Norman, 13–14, 26, 59
Crawford, J., 66, 79
Critical listening, 25
Cultural background: differences caused by, 13;
nonverbal communication and, 22
Cure vs. care, 23

Data: gathering of, 5, 6, 8; in medical interview,
31–38. See also Medical interview
Death: coping with, 24; stages of, 60;
understanding of, 72

De Beauvoir, S., 59, 61
Decision making: by patient, 57; in team health care, 83, 89; with families, 68–69
Deductive organization, 104
Definitions in oral presentations, 106
Demeanor: in oral presentations, 108; of physician, 36
Denotative meaning, 15
Developmental problems in children, 74
Diagnosis, explanation of, 55–56
Diagnostic procedure, explanation of, 56
Discussion as communication skill, 9
Disease vs. illness, 14
Doerfler, D. D., 68, 79
Droge, D., 74, 79
Dunn, K., 40, 46, 68, 79
Dying patient, 58–60

Education, impact of, 13; and patient, 29. See also Conclusion of interview
Emotional problems in children, 74
Empathy, 65
Empathic vs. critical listening, 8
Environment, and nonverbal communication, 18–19
Environmental variables, 6
Erikson, E., 71, 79
Erkko, R., 12, 26
Euphemisms, 42
Examining room procedure, 30
Examples: use of, 40; in presentations, 106
Eye contact, 31; in nonverbal communication, 8, 19; in oral presentations, 108

Facial expression, 8, 18, 21–22; in oral presentations, 108
Fantasy themes, 92
Family: communicating bad news to, 65–66; crises involving, 62; dynamics of, 63; illness management and, 63; providing information to, 67; psychological health and, 62; relieving anxiety of, 65; role of, 62–63, 65
Fass, H. E., 74, 79
Father-husband illness, 68
Fear, 12
Feedback, 16, 50, 92; audiotaping and, 43; with hospitalized patient, 50–51; providing of, 101–102
Fee schedule, 32
Fletcher, C. M., 38, 46
Foley, R., 43, 46
Forming group stage, 90
Francis, V., 75, 79
Frank, J. D., 39, 46
Fritz, P. A., 76, 79

Geiger, Jack, 104, 106, 109
Genital ambiguity, communicating news of, 66
Geriatric patient: communication with, 75–76; expectations of, 76
Gestures, 8, 108
Golden, J. S., 16, 26
Gorton, T. A., 68, 79
Gozzi, E. K., 75, 79
Grant, B. W., 88, 110

Grief, 24
Groups, 82–95; communication in, 93–94; decision making in, 89; development of, 86–87; goals of, 83; language of, 91–92; leadership in, 86–87; meetings of, 94–95; membership roles in, 84–86; norms of, 90–92; physician-nurse relationship in, 87–89. See also Health care team
Guidance-cooperation physician-patient relationship, 28

Halstead, L. S., 82, 110
Health care personnel: as medical team members, 82; physician interaction with, 81–110
Health care system and physician's role in, 4
Health care team, 82–95; communication flow in, 92–95; charting and, 93–94; goals of, 83; interaction of, 95; role responsibilities of, 84–86
Hershman, P. S., 76, 79
History-taking, 29, 30. See also sexual history
Hollender, M. H. A., 28, 47, 49, 51, 61
Homosexuality, 42
Hospital administrator, medical team and, 83
Hospitalized patient, 27, 48–60; acutely ill, 49; bedside manner with, 51–55; communicating information to, 55–58; parent-child relationship and, 50–51; parent-infant relationship and, 50; significant others and, 63; support networks for, 58
Hospital personnel, identification of, 51–52
House of God, 91
Hulka, B. S., 68, 79
Humor, 40
Husband-father illness, 68

Ideas: for oral presentations, 106; organization of, 104
Idioms, 42
Illness: behavior, 68; vs. disease, 14; family patterns producing, 62–63
Inductive organization, 104
Infants: in medical interview, 72; vocabulary development of, 70
Information: clarification of, 97–98; confidentiality of, 59, 67; conveying of, 2, 5, 6, 67; coordination of, 98–99; eliciting of, 33–34; flow of, 92–95; gathering of, 8; for hospitalized patient, 55–58; misinterpretation of, 2; organization of, 9; release of, 77–78; and sexual history, 40–43
Informed consent, 57
Initiative vs. guilt development, 71
Instruction: affect sharing in, 100–101; as communication, 99–102; feedback in, 101–102; lectures as, 102–109; participatory, 100
Instructional materials for patient use, 29
Interactional communication, 18
Interpersonal communication, 6, 13; adult-adult, 28; parent-child, 50–51; parent-infant, 50; vs. charting, 95–96; of medical team, 95
Interpersonal relationships, 13; adult-adult, 28
Interphysician relationships, 95–99; and authority hierarchy, 97; conflicting opinions and, 97–98; referrals in, 96; treatment coordination in, 98–99

Interviews, 31–38. *See also* Medical interview
Introduction, for oral presentations, 103

Jargon, 34, 91; phase, 70
Johansson, R., 12, 26
Johnson, G. D., 16, 26

Kane, J. C., 17, 26
Kinsey, Alfred C., 41
Korsch, B. M., 75, 79
Kubler-Ross, E., 60, 61

Language: choice of, 7; connotative, 16; denotative, 15; development of, 70–75; as health care norm, 91–92; in sexual history taking, 42; simplification of, 16
Larson, R. F., 15, 16, 26
Leader vs. leadership, 87
Leadership: of health care team, 86–87; vs. leader, 87
Lectures, 102–109; audience for, 102–103; conclusion for, 109; deductive organization of, 104; ideas for, 106; inductive organization of, 104; introduction for, 103; presentation of, 107–109; subpoints in, 105; summary statement in, 105; transitions in, 105
Ley, P., 88
Lieberman, M. A., 58, 61
Lipkin, M., 59, 61
Listening, 8, 52; critical, 25; empathic, 8
Litigation, 3–4
Litman, T. J., 68, 79

Mabry, J. H., 68, 80
Malpractice suits, 4, 13
March, V., 57, 61
Marcuse, D. J., 82, 111
"M*A*S*H," 92
May, J. R., 82, 111
Meaning, connotative, 7; denotative, 7
Medical history, 31–38; of children, 69–70; identification of significant others in, 64; sexual information for, 40–43
Medical interview, 31–38; of children, 71, 72–75; conclusion of, 37–38; 45; communication in, 32–33, 44; eliciting information in, 33–34; 44; establishing rapport in, 32, 36–37; maintaining direction of, 34–35, 44; pace of, 35; self-assessment in, 43, 44–45; summary in, 33, 34; vocal cues in, 21–22
Medical office, 29, 31
Medical team. *See* Groups; Health care team
Meyer, D. M., 43, 47
Milmoe, S., 21, 26
Minorities, 13
Misfortune, coping with, 24
Mobilization of family resources, 63
Montgomery, A. B., 43, 47
Morris, D. M., 34, 47
Mother-wife illness, 68
Motivation of patients, 39–40
Mutual participation physician-patient relationship, 28

Nader, P. R., 68, 79
Nagi, S. Z., 81, 110
Nervousness, 21
Network communication, 62–78. *See also* Family; Significant others
Nonsignificant others; communication with, 77
Nonverbal communication, 7–8, 18–23; cultural background and, 22; environmental influences on, 18–19; eye contact as, 19; facial expression as, 21; proxemics and, 19; touch and, 20; vs. verbalization, 22–23; vocal expression in, 21–22. *See also* Verbal communication
Norming group stage, 90
Norms, 90–92; conflict in, 90; dysfunctional, 90
Nukkis, R. V., 57, 61
Nurses, 97; and physician relationship, 87–89

Office environment, 29
Open-ended questioning, 33–34
Oral presentations, 102–109; conclusion of, 37–38; summary of, 105, 109; vividness of, 40; vocal cues in, 108
Organization of information, 9; in medical interview, 35; in oral presentation, 104–105
Osmond, H., 24, 26
Outpatients, 28–46; communication with, 31–38; environmental influences on, 29–31. *See also* Ambulatory patient

Parent-child relationship, 50–51
Parent-infant relationship, 50
Parsons, T., 50, 61
Participatory instruction, 100
Patient(s): ambulatory, 27–46; anger expression by, 21; attitude of, 6, 13, *14, 15;* children as, 69–70; communicating with, 2, 11–25; compliance of, 14; cooperation of, 6; definition of, 12; demeanor of, 18; dignity of, 53; dying role of, 24; educational background of, 1, 13 *14;* expectations of, 32; families of, 62–79; fears of, 12, 23; geriatric, 75–76; hospitalized, 27, 48–60; interviews of, 31–38; management of, 10; misunderstandings of, 1, 6; motivating of, 39; outpatients, 64; as participants in care, 4; and physician relationship, 18–23; privacy of, 54; receptivity of, 39–40; referrals of, 96; role expectations of, 13–14, 20, 32, 37; scheduling of, 29–30; shy, 35; sick role of, 24; significant others and, 63; stress factors affecting, 18–19; support networks for, 58–69; technology and, 49; verbose, 35. *See also* Family; Significant others
Patient advocates, 76
Patient rights groups, 4
Pediatrician-patient relationship, 72–75
Pediatric patient, 69–75
Performing group stage, 90
Personalization of physician-patient relationship, 52–53
Personal presentation, 9, 108
Personal space, 19
Persuasive communication, 39–40
Phillips, G. M., 105, 110
Physical examination, 37, 45

Physician(s), 12; attitude of, 14; coordination among, 95–96; as manager, 10; as medical team leader, 86–87; and nurse relationship, 87–89; office of, 29, 30; and patient relationship, 4, 5, 12, 54; roles of, 7, 50; as support giver, 23; traditional model of, 16; vocabulary of, 15
Piaget, J., 71, 80; developmental stages of, 71–72
Pomeroy, W. B., 42, 47
Posture, 8
Pratt, I., 69, 80
Presentations, 102–109. *See also* Lectures
Primary authority in treatment, 96–97
Privacy, 32; for hospitalized patient, 54
Problem solving, 5, 6. *See also* Decision making
Process-centered roles, 84
Proxemics, 19
Psychosocial development, 71
Psychosomatic illness, 63

Questioning, 8; vs. participation, 100; for patient interviews, 33–34; in sexual history taking, 41–42

Rae-Grant, Q. A. F., 82, 111
Rapport, 33; with ambulatory patient, 36, 45; physicial examination and, 37; with hospitalized patient, 51–55; physician-patient, 33
Reading, A., 14, 26
Referrals, 96, 98
Requests, 96
Roles: clarification of, 85; conflicts of, 86; flexibility of, 7; of health care team, 84–86; modeling of, 99–100; of patient, 24
Rosenthal, R., 21, 26
Rowland, I. P., 15, 26
Rubin, I. M., 86, 87, 90
Russell, C. G., 76, 79
Rutala, P. J., 43, 47

Samara, J., 15, 16, 26
Saunders, L., 15, 16, 26
Seating arrangements, 30
Selective perception, 25
Self-assessment for medical interview, 43, 44t–45t
Self-help groups, 4, 13
Senior, B., 39, 47
Separation anxiety, 71
Settings, of physician-patient relationship, 18–19, 29–32, 48–55
Severely ill patient, 58–60
Sex, discussion of, 41
Sexual history, 40–43
Sharf, B. F., 43, 46
Shem, S., 91, 111
Shy patients, 35
Sick role, 50
Siebert, S., 37, 47
Siegler, M., 24, 26
Significant others, 63, 64; identification of, 64–65; role of, 68–69
Situational adaptation, 7–8
Situational analysis, 6–7
Smilansky, J., 110
Smith, B. A., 39, 47

Spatial distance, 8
Speaker, physician as, 102–109
Speech, development of, 70
Spellman, M. S., 88, 110
Spock, B., 107
Starfield, B., 37, 47
Statistics in oral presentations, 106
Status differences, 12
Stein, L. I., 88, 111
Steinwachs, D., 37, 47
Stillman, P. L., 43, 47
Stoeckle, J. D., 34, 47
Storming group stage, 90
Stranger anxiety, 71
Stress, 19
Subpoint organization, 105
Supportive behavior, 23–26
Support network, 58–60
Sutton-Smith, K., 57, 61
Sympathetic vs. empathic behavior, 25
Szasz, T. S., 28, 47, 49, 51, 61

Task accomplishment. *See also* Process-centered roles
Team health care, 82. *See also* Health care team
Technology, 81; patient response to, 49
Tension, minimizing of, 42
Toddler: in medical interview, 72; vocabulary development of, 70
Topics for oral presentations, 104
Touch, 8; in nonverbal communication, 20
Transition statements, 105
Treatment: coordination of, 98–99; explanation of, 56; family's role in, 68–69
Trust: vs. distrust, 71; securing of, 32
Tubesing, N. L., 89, 111
Tuchman, B. W., 90, 111
Tyroler, H. A., 68, 79

Vanderpool, N. A., 40, 46, 68, 79
Veach, T. L., 43, 47
Verbal communication, 22–23. *See also* Nonverbal communication
Verbose patient, 35
Videotaping: of interviews, 43. *See also* Educational materials, 29
Visual aids, 40; in oral presentations, 108
Vocabulary: development of, 70; jargon in, 91; medical, 15
Vocal cues, 8; in oral presentations, 108; with patients, 21–22
Voice intonation, 8; pitch, 8; tone, 8
Vuori, H., 12, 26

Waiting room procedure, 29
Westin, C., 37, 47
Wiens, A., 42, 47
Wife-mother illness, 68
Wilcox, E. M., 76, 79
Wish, J. B., 91, 111
Wolk, I., 21, 26
Words as symbols, 15

Zollen, J. J., 105, 110